I0759398

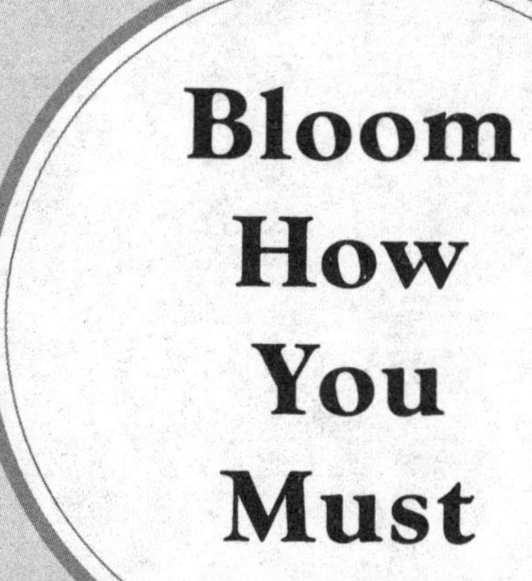
Bloom
How
You
Must

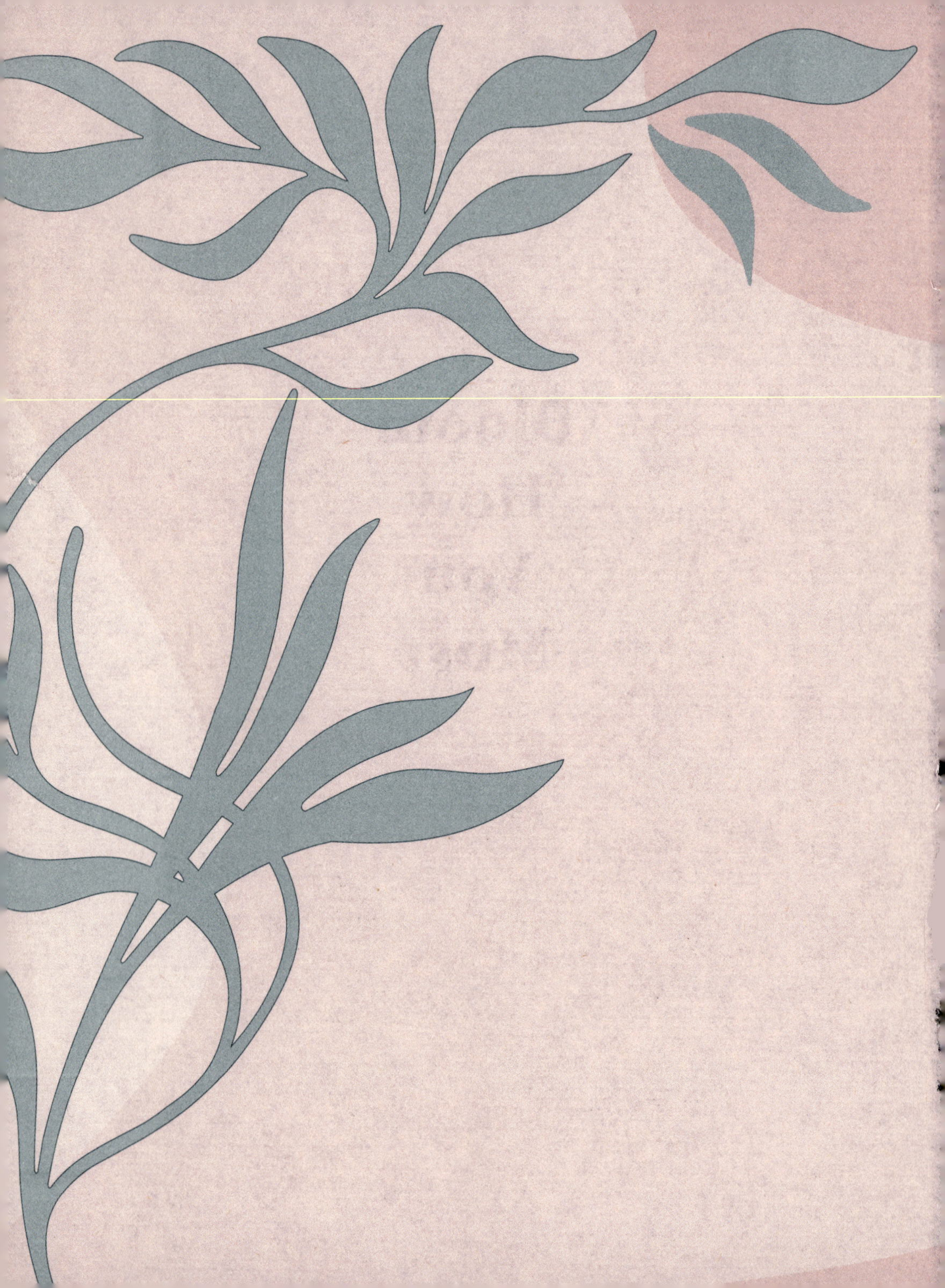

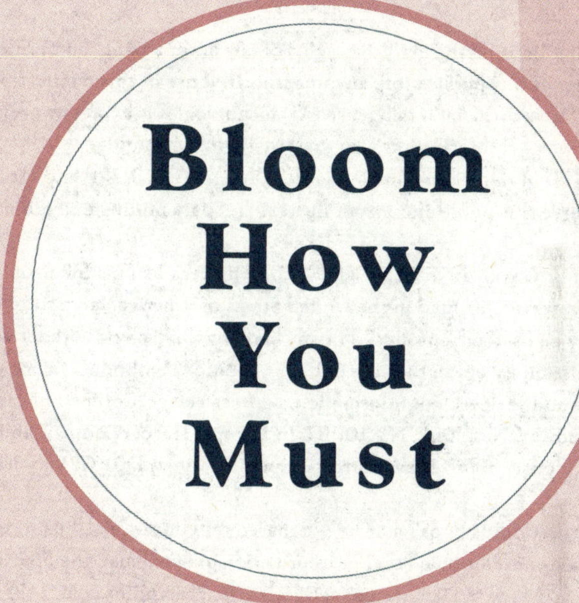

Bloom How You Must

A BLACK WOMAN'S GUIDE TO SELF-CARE AND GENERATIONAL HEALING

TARA PRINGLE JEFFERSON

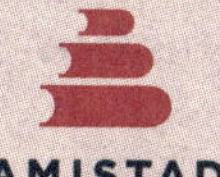

AMISTAD

An Imprint of HarperCollins*Publishers*

HarperCollins books may be purchased for educational, business, or sales promotional use. For information, please email the Special Markets Department at SPsales@harpercollins.com.

FIRST EDITION

harpercollins.com

Designed by Bonni Leon-Berman

Library of Congress Cataloging-in-Publication Data has been applied for.

ISBN 978-0-06-337787-5

25 26 27 28 29 LBC 5 4 3 2 1

CONTENTS

Black Wellness Matters

More than a decade ago, before I dedicated most of my waking hours to being a self-care coach, I was a 26-year-old mother of two, working insanely long hours as a freelance consultant and writer after an unexpected bout of unemployment due to the Great Recession.

I was regularly pulling eighteen-hour days working from my dining room table, rotating different types of eye drops to soothe my vision instead of addressing the real issue—too much screen time. My husband would come home from work to find me hunched over the computer, the same position I was in when he left for the day. And the same position I would be in when he went upstairs for bed.

After nearly a year of this pace, one day I woke up with pain in my neck and shoulder. I figured I just slept wrong, so I took a couple ibuprofen and kept working.

But then the next day, certain areas on my neck were warm to the touch and very painful. Again, I chalked it up to a night of tossing and turning. I figured I'd give it one more day and then I'd go get it checked out.

The next morning came and the pain greeted me as I opened my eyes. I had been alternating heat and cold on my shoulder for the past two days and no relief. Now my ears were ringing and I had no idea what was causing it.

As symptoms piled up, I decided to go to urgent care that Friday. I'll note that I waited until after I dropped my kids off at school. The doctor, a slim woman in her mid-forties, sat on the stool and looked at me expectantly. "What brings you in today?"

I gave her a rundown of my issues and she began to give a head-to-toe exam, uncovering new issues at every turn.

She took my temperature. "Oh, it's a little high. Do you feel warm?"

"No."

"Do you feel like you're coming down with something?"

"Um, no."

She took my blood pressure. "Oh, your blood pressure is slightly elevated. Is that normal?"

"No." *Blood pressure is high too?*

"Well, perhaps you're coming down with something?"

"Maybe," I replied, feeling a bit sheepish that I seemed to be falling apart on this exam table.

She examined my ears. "Oh, you have a bit of redness there. I can tell there's some fluid buildup in your ears—it's pressing on your eardrum, which is probably causing the ringing."

"Okay."

She examined my neck, pressing and asking if anything hurt. Before I could answer, she frowned and rubbed a spot under my jaw. "You have a swollen lymph node here."

That's what that is, I thought to myself.

She stepped back and gave me a pity smile, as she sat down on her stool. I rubbed my hands together and waited.

She ran down my treatment plan and I nodded, ready to get out of there and get back to work. I had a work deadline that I absolutely could not miss. I just wanted to get my prescription and go.

As she finished her instructions, her face turned serious. "I want you to rest this weekend."

I nodded and began to slide off the exam table, half listening as I gathered my things.

"No, I mean it." She held her hand up to slow me down. "It's obvious you are doing too much when you can't even slow down to notice how your body feels. I want you to go home, get in the bed, and not get out until Monday. Do you understand? Take it easy this weekend."

It wasn't until I got to the car that I realized the doctor had just given me *a literal prescription to rest.* A permission slip to take two full days to rest my body and give myself time and attention that I had obviously been lacking.

I was only 26 but I was already working myself to death.

I had no reason to suspect that my pace was unsustainable. I have grown up watching Black women at large be exhausted as a matter of principle. As far back as I can see in my family tree, women worked hard, provided for their families, and made change in their communities. We would always do what needed to be done, no matter how our minds, bodies, or spirits felt.

In the years that followed that fateful doctor's appointment, I wondered out loud: *How did our mothers do this? Our grandmothers? How did they manage to stay grounded and care for themselves while also living under oppressive conditions? How did they find joy for themselves in a society determined to snuff it out?*

What is it, I wondered, *that keeps Black women whole?*

HOW WE MAKE IT THROUGH

THE QUICK ANSWER is that often Black women are not whole. We are mighty, but we're human. Our minds and bodies often tell the story when we cannot tell it for ourselves. Black women are 60 percent more likely to be diagnosed with high blood pressure.[1] Black people get less restorative sleep than any other racial group[2] and are more likely to report symptoms of mental distress,[3] with fewer community resources or Black mental health professionals in place to help us navigate. Research has shown that the consistent effects of stress can lead to what is known in the medical field as "weathering," meaning Black women are, on average, biologically 7.5 years older than our white counterparts.[4]

Nearly every book or research study I've read on Black women in the past few years has given a damn near identical litany of stats to let us know our well-being is in a state of emergency.

But perhaps there was something I missed. With all the words used to describe Black women, *exhausted* can't be all we are.

Right?

I began to slow down in my personal and professional life. As you'll read in later chapters, that slowdown undoubtedly saved my life. When I took a step back, I was able to discover that just as Black women have a legacy of strength and resilience, we also have a legacy of self-care that often goes unpraised and underreported.

Look into the memoirs and stories of any number of notable Black women and you'll see glimpses of our self-care legacy there. In her posthumous memoir, *Coretta: My Life, My Love, My Legacy,* Coretta Scott King recalled her come-to-Jesus conversation with her husband, Martin Luther King Jr.: "I love being your wife and the mother of your children but if that's all I am to do, I'll go crazy." She was determined to carve out her own lane and used her gifts as a singer to support the movement. Toward the end of her life, she took a few trips with good friends Betty Shabazz, widow of Malcolm X, and Myrlie Evers-Williams, widow of Medgar Evers. The trio offered each other a particular sisterhood. When they were together, their main goal was to "enjoy not being in charge of anything," King wrote.

Toni Morrison spent time with the earth, using it to clear her mind long enough to give us works like *The Bluest Eye* and *Beloved.* While raising two children as a single working mother, she grew hearty vegetables and beautiful flowers. One of her most prized possessions was a four-foot-wide jade bush she grew from a cutting of a jade plant belonging to Nelson Mandela. She loved birds and had her own tactics for keeping her property clear of bird droppings: "Take a shotgun, and when you see the birds come close, shoot a couple of rounds into the air," she told *Audubon* magazine. "Only a few rounds though and never directly at the birds. This lets them know that they are not to shit on your space anymore. This is your space now." (A lesson on boundaries if I ever heard one.)

Nothing much separates these women from the women in our

own family history. This book, filled with the voices of "regular" Black women, from their late teens to their nineties, is a reminder to you that we're not new to this.

We're true to this.

This self-care inheritance gets passed down from generation to generation, in ways seen and unseen. It's time we take it out of the shadows and allow it to bloom in the light.

LET'S TALK LEGACY

IN THE SELF CARE SUITE, we host small, intimate gatherings to discuss everything from pleasure to creativity to relationships. No matter the topic, I always begin each event the same way, asking attendees, "Who taught you how to take care of yourself, for better or worse?"

We start with those "seeds" of their own lived reality—what did they witness among the adults in their lives? What lessons, both spoken and unspoken, seeped through to their subconsciousness?

The women usually go silent as they think of their answer. Then one by one, they'll raise their hand and give me a story about their mother:

"She never left the house without her hair done."

"She had houseplants everywhere—you couldn't walk through a room without seeing four or five plants in the corner. She'd sing to them in the mornings."

"She'd take a nap every Sunday after church and made sure the whole house had to be quiet!"

Sometimes they'll tell a story about their grandmother or an aunt. Nine times out of ten, their self-care legacy always comes back to a maternal figure. That relationship (or lack thereof) informs how well they take care of themselves today.

Inevitably, one attendee will say that no one taught her. "I can't think of a single example," she'll say. "They were really horrible at taking care of themselves. All they did was work and then come home to take care of us."

I insist that, too, is a lesson. Sometimes that self-care legacy is less of a roar and more of a whisper, a reminder that a life dedicated to the pursuit of happiness was not on the table for many of our foremothers. That walk down memory lane is a glimpse into the small ways Black women have sustained themselves through personal turmoil and societal strife.

Granted, our foremothers weren't walking around calling those little sips of leisure "self-care." They were just trying to find wholeness however they could. Stress and exhaustion are not new concepts; our language today is just different. Instead of being depressed, they might have simply "been in a bad way." Instead of being anxious, they might have said, "My nerves are bad." (Shout out to Dr. Angela Neal-Barnett's 2001 anxiety handbook, *Soothe Your Nerves*, for this link between language and lineage.)

Part of our legacy is not just that we've survived, but *how* we've survived.

BLOOM HOW YOU MUST

IN MY NETWORK, conversations about self-care reached a fever pitch in the aftermath of the 2016 presidential election and in the years that followed. Suddenly, everyone was grasping for something to steady them in an increasingly unstable world. People who teased me for my "woo-woo stuff" in prior years suddenly wanted to know if I could recommend a yoga class or if I had a favorite brand of weighted blankets.

I watched history repeat itself after the results of the 2024 election rolled in. People were again dedicating themselves to notions of comfort and community. *What can I do, where can I go that feels good?* Always a reminder that self-care is not a trend, but a matter of fortification when the world surprises or disappoints, as it often does.

Don't get me wrong. Self-care alone does not solve these complex societal issues. A good meditation session or a good nap is incredible, but it's not going to cure all that ails us. That's the job of progressive policy that puts Black women's health and well-being at the center. But my question is: *What are Black women going to do in the meantime? How do we weather the difficulties that come with living in an anti-Black society with some sense of calm and strength?*

Skeptics and critics contend that self-care (in its limited definition) can't be sufficient and sustaining, especially for women of color. One such critic, Toronto-based community organizer Nakita Valerio, went viral with her quote, "Shouting 'self-care' at people who actually need 'community care' is how we fail people.

"Self-care does not address the systemic issue that people who face compounded discrimination have to deal with," Valerio told Mashable.[5] "I might be getting a pedicure but it's not going to stop someone from coming up to me and asking me why I'm wearing a hijab. I'm Muslim. We [Muslim women] can't just leave our identity at home when we go and get our pedicures."

I'm a huge believer of community care in all its forms: mutual aid, babysitting swaps, meal trains, and so on. As a Black woman, I wouldn't be writing this book if I didn't believe in using our voice and energy to uplift and care for other Black women. In fact, this book wouldn't be possible without community care.

I'll push back on the debate between community care and self-care only slightly by reminding you, dear reader, *there is no either/or.* There is no need to apply scarcity to the idea that Black women can only receive or request care one way.

We need both.

Both exist in harmony. If I am run ragged and have not taken a moment to collect myself, what do I have to offer my community? If I haven't secured my own mask, as flight attendants instruct us to do in moments of crisis, then how can I expect to be of any help to others? We must each be recipients of the care we need, without question or hesitation.

I want a world where Black women are catered to, loved on, studied, included, protected. I want a world where we have a surplus of people asking (daily!), "What do you need, sis? How is your heart? What can I do for you?"

And even in *that* world, we would still need to be able to answer. Knowing what we need is a key component of self-care and will never shift to become someone else's responsibility.

As Black women, we are the blueprint for community care. The bonding and psychology of hair salons, the women's groups that organized for some of the political rights we enjoy today, the way Black women represent over and over at the ballot box—we know how to show up for each other.

There's nothing more radical than deciding to show up for ourselves. Our collective depends on it. If we want a better future, it starts with being rested and nourished and cared for. As Angela Davis said, "Anyone who's interested in making a change in the world, also has to learn how to take care of herself, himself, theirselves."[6]

I want to remind us all that oppression and discrimination are not all we are. We do ourselves a disservice when we view ourselves solely through the lens of what this violent society does to us.

In 90 percent of the interviews I've done, I'm asked to define self-care. And each time I come up with a slightly different answer, depending on what I've been reading and how my thinking has evolved over time.

One part of the definition that has never wavered is that *self-care is a personal commitment to the actions that lift your spirit, soothe your mind, and care for your body.* It can be as simple as asking what you need and then figuring out how to give it to yourself. It's this simple framework that I urge Black women to cling to.

Self-care allows us to reclaim our humanity, to insist that all parts of our lives matter and we deserve the space and energy to nurture ourselves in whatever way we see fit. Self-care is a way for us to reclaim our agency, to give ourselves permission to slow down and take a deep breath. Self-care is but one tool for us to be gentle with ourselves, to understand how we can navigate any given situation with care and concern for our own well-being as paramount.

What a concept for Black women.

Critics are often careful to draw a line between "real" self-care and the "fluffy" stuff. But even still, "fluffy" self-care has its place. For a woman working two jobs and raising two kids, that one hour she spends on her nails might be the thing that she looks forward to at the end of a long week, the way she chooses to express herself. I've learned that I cannot judge what self-care looks like for other women.

Your own self-care practice is yours to define, shape, and overhaul. You can go as deep as you want, exploring those parts of yourself that need tending. It may look different from moment to moment, from season to season. What you need now might be different once you fast-forward five years.

A self-care practice is just that—something you *practice*. You won't always be even-keeled and happy and stress-free. Life will get a little messy and stressful from time to time. But more often than not, a solid self-care practice will keep you close to your source and expand your reserves so you can tend to the corners of your life without succumbing to exhaustion day after day. And while we can't control those larger societal forces, we can use our awareness of them to build—to the best of our ability—sustaining habits and rituals that give us our best shot at a life of ease and happiness.

Ease is the most radical concept I can think of. Going back generations, the women in my family only know hard work, showing up even when you're dog-tired. There is always *something else to do.* The to-do list is never ending because it goes back to what your mama and her mama couldn't get to.

OUR ORIGINS

FOR THE VERY first event of The Self Care Suite, I hosted a two-day retreat in Alexandria, Virginia. I was new to the wellness game but I knew two things for certain: Women desperately needed an affordable getaway and they needed someone to give them permission to snatch their happiness with both hands.

In our second session, Washington, DC–based therapist Esther

Boykin tasked the women with adopting a more aggressive approach to self-care. In other words, choosing to do the completely selfish thing every once in a while.

Most attendees sat thoughtfully and nodded, scribbling notes on their hotel stationery. But one sat uncomfortably, shaking her head.

"I . . . can't do that," she said. She had five children, three from a previous marriage and two from her husband's previous marriage. She was all about that blended family life and being as present as possible for her family. At this point in her life, *mother* was her primary identity.

"That's just not what a good mother does," she continued, tears beginning to flow. "How can I just leave them and do something for me when they need stuff? I've been doing this [motherhood] for a long time. It just . . . doesn't sound like what a good mother does. I can't do that."

The room went silent as the attendee sobbed quietly, her friend giving her a two-arm embrace as she sat with her feelings.

Boykin paused thoughtfully and let the tears land. (Amen for booking therapists who know how to handle the heavy moments!)

"Could you consider a reframe?" she asked gently. "Is that how you want your daughter to experience motherhood? Could you consider what it means to your daughter to see you taking time for yourself?"

The attendee nodded and wiped her face. "I will think about that."

Sometime after that same friend left the retreat, she went home and challenged herself: She'd commit to Friday night outings where she'd meet with a friend for dinner or take herself out to the movies on a solo date.

Progress.

In taking a stand and committing ourselves to a life less laborious, we end up doing the hard work of shifting a bloodline. As my friend Natalyn Bradshaw suggests: *Who shifts when you shift? Who heals when you do? Who changes when you change?*

CLAIM YOUR LEGACY

IN ASKING WOMEN, "Who taught you how to take care of yourself?" sometimes they turn the question back on me before I can blink.

My answer goes back to three Black women over three generations—Marilyn (my mom), Louise (my paternal grandmother), and Marietta (my maternal grandmother).

My mother was and still is one of the most hands-on mothers I've ever seen, and now that I'm a mother myself I wonder how she had the energy for three young girls, a full-time job, and nursing school.

Except sometimes she didn't have the energy.

Every so often, maybe once a year or so, my mother would reach her limit. She was stressed and tired and in need of a break. She'd pack a bag and plan to spend the weekend at a nearby hotel, eating room service and sleeping until noon, leaving my dad to tend to the three of us for a night or two.

But every so often she'd call home and ask my dad to bring us up to the hotel because she missed us. And we would come, bringing our loud and boisterous selves all up in her relaxation space. From her example I learned (for better or worse) that *being a mother is all-encompassing and that sacrifice is the name of the game.*

I spent a good chunk of summers as a child with my grandmother Louise, in Buffalo, New York. Her two-bedroom house was small but always tidy. My two sisters and I spent many days watching my grandmother be a one-woman tornado, always flitting around moving from one room to the next, from one store to the next. We had errands to run and meals to prepare. *Idleness?* Louise did not know her. It wasn't until I was maybe 11 years old that I saw my grandmother be horizontal. (Watching five grandkids under 11 for a week straight was the only situation to take her down.) I honestly didn't think she needed sleep. I figured she ran on something otherworldly that the rest of us couldn't access. She was always awake, no matter what time we went to bed or rose in the morning. Once my sister told me she woke up thirsty at two in the morning, and when she went into the kitchen, Louise was there, at the kitchen table, ready to get her a glass of water and shoo her back to bed. From her example I learned (for better or worse) that tending to your family takes work and consistency. *You are expected to always be on.*

On the flip side, my newborn homecoming was to a house directly across the street from my maternal grandmother. By the time I was born, Marietta was a widowed 65-year-old retiree. She was happy to serve as our de facto babysitter, which meant I spent tons of nights and weekends feeling safe and protected in her two-family home in East Cleveland, Ohio.

Every day at noon, right after *The Price Is Right* but before the soaps, my grandmother would summon all three of us into her full-size bed, tuck us in under a heavy blanket no matter the season, and command us to rest for a minimum of one hour.

To this day I get inexplicably tired at 11:55 a.m.

Surely this was a 70-year-old woman's ploy to get some rest herself in the middle of the day. On those days when we were too wound up to nap correctly—quietly and remaining in bed—she would lie on the outer boundary of the mattress, using her body as a soft, warm barrier between us and playtime. *Now,* she'd instruct us, *it's time to rest.* Even as a teen, when I was far past the midday nap routine you usually associate with toddlers, she'd pat the blanket and expect me to get in. So I did.

When I woke up an hour or so later, usually sticky with sweat, she'd be in her favorite chair that straddled the living room and dining room, chuckling at her stories and feeling ready for the second half of her shift as babysitter.

In her way, she was offering a lesson—*power down sometimes.* You can't run yourself into the ground, no matter how helpful you want to be. It doesn't escape me that my most enduring lessons on rest came from the eldest member of my family, a full generation ahead of my paternal grandmother. She had learned to lean into the ease that age brings.

This is my self-care legacy. There's more work than rest but *rest is there.*

On my own way to wellness, I've had to work through the lessons they've subconsciously taught me. *Do I need to be the first person in my house to wake each day? Am I allowed to cry in front of my children? Does the world stop spinning if I don't make dinner every night? Can I take a mental health day or is that lazy?*

Interrogating that blueprint you were handed is the first step to making it your own.

As you start, you might realize that you have not personally witnessed your mother or grandmother or aunts prioritize themselves in any way that is recognizable. You may have witnessed them wake before the sun, prepare meals that everybody requested and enjoyed, clean the house, work that job, and encourage you to do the same, whether spoken or unspoken.

And if that's your legacy, and it's wearing you thin, it's even more reason for you to take the lead and begin a new one for your lineage.

EXAMINE YOUR OWN BELIEFS

HOW CAN WE know where we're going if we don't know where we've been? Or, as my good sis Lauryn Hill would say, "How you gon' win if you ain't right within?"

Our own beliefs about self-care didn't just form overnight, but are the result of years of observation and experience. These "seeds" were presented to you, and at some point they began to make up your primary inner dialogue. Again, I ask: *Who taught you?*

If we don't start here, meaningful additions and changes to your self-care practice will likely fall flat.

To start you off, here are the ten questions I ask women as they begin to interrogate their self-care beliefs:

- Who raised you?
- Who did you spend the majority of your time with growing up?
- Who was influential in your formative years (teachers, siblings, family members)?
- Who looked "happy" to you?
- Who looked like they were just barely getting by?

- Did your parents/guardians have any self-care rituals that you can identify now?
- As a child, what did you do to soothe yourself when you were upset or frustrated?
- Was there any discussion of mental/emotional health growing up?
- What images from media (TV/movies/music) do you remember that shaped how you feel about self-care?
- How have your ideas on self-care shifted over time?

REMEMBER THAT THESE questions—particularly the first six—aren't meant to be answered with judgment. There are no right or wrong answers here. Fight any inclination to assign blame or shame. We're simply tilling the soil and assessing our foundation. Spending time here helps us later when we're working to make significant changes in how we care for ourselves.

SEVEN PILLARS OF SELF-CARE

I'M WILLING TO bet that when most people think of self-care, they're thinking of physical health—going to the doctor, eating fruits and vegetables, and making sure you're drinking enough water. (Let this be a quick reminder for you to go drink some water.)

But true wellness encompasses so much more than your physical self. That's why you might have found yourself exhausted in the morning after a full night's rest. If you're feeling unheard in your relationships or unsatisfied at work, a nap or a massage might not be the fix.

Emily and Amelia Nagoski, authors of *Burnout: The Secret to Unlocking the Stress Cycle*, gave one of the best definitions of wellness I've read:

> To be well is not to live in a state of perpetual safety and calm, but to move fluidly from a state of adversity, risk, adventure or excitement, back to safety and calm, and out again. Stress is not bad for you; being stuck is bad for you. Wellness happens when your body is a place of safety for you, even when your body is not necessarily in a safe place. You can be well, even during the times when you don't feel good.[7]

Wellness isn't a static goal where once we achieve it we live happily ever after. It's about being able to ride the ebbs and flows of life with more confidence, more vigor, more enthusiasm!

Let's learn to create a life of holistic wellness, where we build ourselves up in six different dimensions. We will examine each of these in depth, to help you hone in on roadblocks and turn them into new habits:

Physical wellness is tending to your physical body to aid in rest, recovery, and repair for optimal functioning.

Social wellness is investing time into relationships that nourish, uplift, and teach us more about ourselves and the world around us.

Professional wellness is having your gifts and talents affirmed in a space where you are paid appropriately for your time and energy.

Spiritual wellness is understanding your place in the universe and connection to other living beings.

Mental/emotional wellness is knitting our thoughts and emotions together for a more positive outlook, deepening mental health reserves, and practicing vulnerability to share with a trusted community.

Creative wellness is being able to flex your creative muscles in a way that satisfies and brings out the divine in you.

Now that you have a good sense of what each facet of wellness entails, take a few minutes to run through this self-care inventory to see how you stack up against your ideal. Every item won't be applicable to you and your goals so there is no traditional "scoring." Instead, you are measuring *Current You* against *Future You*. Where would she like to be and how can you get her there?

Your Wellness Quiz

On an average day I get about _____ to myself to use however I choose:

Less than an hour

One to two hours

More than two hours

I frequently feel unfocused during the day.

Exactly this. Nearly every day.

At times, yes.

Nah, I've done pretty well with my focus this past year!

I am constantly rushing from one activity to the next.

All. The. Time.

Sometimes.

Nah, my pace has slowed a bit over the past year.

My brain is operating at _____.

100%—I am at max capacity.

75%—My life is feeling mighty full these days.

50%—My life is feeling manageable.

I often cope with stressors by:

Um, not dealing with them. I feel like I might explode.

Getting a release every once in a while.

Having a few tools (meditation, breathing, reaching out to a friend) that keep me balanced.

I am often self-critical.

I can't help it. My inner voice is kinda mean.

Sometimes, when I make mistakes, I get critical.

I've got a pretty good internal script. I'm kind to myself.

I currently exist at the intersection of _____.

Busy and busier.

Finding some balance and energy.

Rest and renewal.

I have cultivated a spiritual practice that encourages and strengthens me.

Eh? Not really.

It's in progress.

I can confidently say yes.

I feel connected to my purpose.

Still trying to figure out what my purpose is.

Some days? Yes.

Yes, I know what I'm here to do!

My gratitude practice is:

Nonexistent.

Inconsistent.

Consistent.

I can trust my intuition.

I've ignored my gut too many times to count.

I tend to second-guess myself.

I've learned to listen when my gut says something!

I have identified muses who inspire me to live creatively.

A muse? Hmm . . . let me think about that.

I think I have one or two.

Yes! My muses help me see life differently.

My wardrobe is full of clothes I like to wear and look cute in.

Oh, I need a whole new wardrobe.

I could use a bit of a refresh.

I do a good job rotating in pieces that feel like me.

I can name three things I like to do for fun that don't involve TV, social media, or another person.

Yikes, three? Nah.

Hmm . . . maybe one or two?

I can name three!

I often feel inspired to create something.

Unless it's creating more time in the day . . . not really.

I dabble a bit in the creative arts.

I spend significant time thinking and moving creatively.

My sleep quality is:

Inconsistent and inefficient.

Better some days than others.

Consistently pretty good.

My libido is in line with what I personally desire.

Nah, it's been MIA and I hate it.

It's been coming and going (ha!).

She is here and accounted for!

I indulge in some form of movement (walking, biking, yoga) most days per week.

Movement is hard to come by—I don't typically get enough in each week.

It varies but I know I could get more.

I'm pretty good at getting in enough movement to help my body feel good.

As I scan my body right now, I can identify:

My body is all knotted up!

There's some tension in my neck/shoulders/hips/legs.

My body feels pretty good.

I struggle with making requests, especially when it comes to asking for help, assistance, or nurturing from others.

I rarely ask people for help.
I can do it depending on the ask.
I try to ask when I really need help.

My quality time with friends over the past year has been:

On the decline.
About the same.
On an upswing.

I've developed a supportive community that helps me feel good to be me.

Whew, no.
I've got a decent crew but it could be stronger.
I feel blessed by my community—they hold me down!

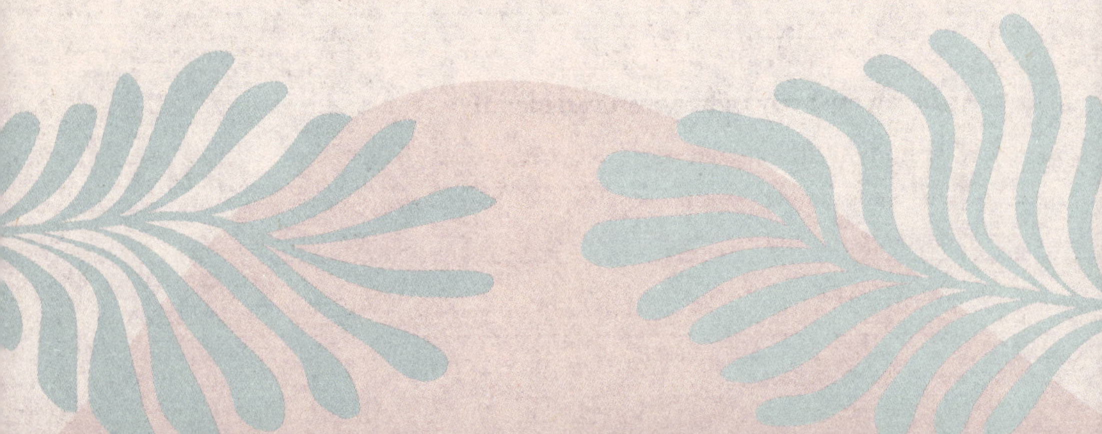

NOW IT'S TIME TO DIVE IN

EARLIER I ASKED myself, *What is it that keeps Black women whole?*

The simplest answer: Black women have kept Black women whole.

Case in point: Most of my life I believed I had a "black thumb." Over the years I tried to grow herbs, veggies, small plants, and without fail, they'd wither and die before they could get going. Even small grocery store arrangements seemed to droop and fall within days.

Clearly I was doing something wrong but I couldn't figure out what it was. Then I joined a Black Girls with Gardens group online and witnessed women having extraordinary success with the plants in their space.

I stopped feeling hopeless. I watched. I asked questions.

I learned I was watering too much in some cases; in others I was watering too little. I was trying to treat each plant the same, not realizing they each had their own individual needs. I didn't realize placing plants in my north-facing windows meant most would wilt from lack of sun.

Ladies in the group taught me I would do well with snake plants, pothos, and jade. I needed to move some houseplants to a different space in the home, repot some others with more coarse soil for drainage. I went from having zero plants to more than forty, all thriving.

It was Black women in my life who showed me the beauty in caring for plants. The practice is about slowing down long enough to know what to look for and how to develop a care plan that ensures the plants have what they need to thrive.

It is this same guidance I'm offering you in this book.

We will do as nature demands when it's time to grow. We will survey the land, analyzing whether the conditions are right for what we're trying to achieve. We sort our seeds, plucking the old and planting the new. We make sure we provide what's necessary to bring it from seed to sprout—water, sun, fertilizer. We inspect invasive weeds and yank them out at the root to stop them from choking out our progress.

When we approach our wellness with the care and precision of a gardener, everything will bloom as it is designed to.

Each chapter intertwines to concoct the ultimate recipe for holistic wellness. You can't have social wellness without emotional support to help you nurture those life-giving relationships. Creative interests bring out your spiritual energy. Your physical self thrives when you tend to the mental stuff and vice versa. You grow as a professional when you get grounded in the truth of who you are and take all these areas of wellness into account. They all marry together and when simmered on low, it makes a delicious gumbo.

SPENDING TIME IN THE GARDEN

FROM THE ONSET, I knew this book needed to include the voices of Black women from all walks of life. This was a collective effort, a challenge to capture the stories of our shared self-care legacies and how we have not only survived but thrived during moments of personal struggle and societal pain. These are the stories we need to share. Loudly. Often.

As I began to shape what would eventually turn into *Bloom How*

You Must, I set about interviewing one hundred Black women, ages 19 to 99.

I call them the Gardeners. I didn't know how long it would take to capture their stories, but I knew that a simple conversation—starting with "Who taught you how to take care of yourself?"—had been the catalyst for my work stretching back over a decade. It would be nourishing, personally, as I cleared room in my schedule and laughed with countless women over Zoom, in coffee shops and churches, and on park benches.

I've interviewed yoga instructors, professors, podcasters, nutritionists, authors. Each gave me a story that reaffirmed the breadth of our experience. Our creativity was on full display as they each recalled a caregiver showing them the ropes in ways they hoped to emulate, or as they detailed how they created their wellness routines from scratch. I wanted a multigenerational look at our experiences, making sure to spread out my focus to those elders.

As an elder millennial, it would have been easy to ground this book in my generational perspective, but this book would not be complete if I did not sit at the feet of older Black women and just listen. Their generational lens focused on hard work, caregiving, and strength. In their minds, taking space for themselves to simply *be* themselves was a liberating concept. The mingling of generations holds the magic sauce, as it allows the younger generations to see the sacrifices made for them and the older generations to relax into the idea of self-advocacy.

One sobering realization: Black women, after a certain age, feel invisible. *Me? You want to talk to me?*

I do, I assured them. Their next question: *Why?* They wondered what about their lives drew me to them. And I was honest: I want to hear from "regular" Black women. The ones you pass at the grocery store, at the post office, at the gym. Their stories reminded me how much beauty you can find in sitting with a stranger. With more than a hundred interviews, this book was not going to fit all of them, but even if you don't see their names, know that their lives informed the work. At the end of each interview, after I double- and triple-checked that my recording was sound, I blew a soft exhale and said the exact same thing out loud to no one in particular: "That was beautiful."

They confirmed what I already knew: that as Black women, we are trying our best to make it in a world that often doesn't offer us much in the way of support. We endure and we stretch. We tend to others far more than we tend to ourselves. We maintain, even in the midst of turmoil and stress, an immense sense of gratitude and resilience. Even among those with no ties to organized religion, we maintain a strong sense of faith in something, even if it is just faith in each other. We often learned this from our mothers, who learned from their mothers, who learned from theirs.

Even if the Gardeners didn't spell it out explicitly, strength is the through line from generation to generation. They praised their mothers for being hardworking and indefatigable. Whatever she did, they told me, she did it well. These mothers cooked and cleaned up after large families, often solo. They insisted on good manners and education. They worked hard, from sunup to sundown.

Perhaps not surprisingly, when I asked about their mothers' leisure time, there were far fewer examples. Most often it was a dedication to church or a strong reliance on a good group of girlfriends that offered space to breathe and collect their thoughts. Community, in all its forms, continues to save us, again and again, generation after generation.

If there was one unanimous opinion, it's this: We have been taught, consciously or unconsciously, that our life is about others. We have learned, by virtue of being a Black woman in this country, that you are supposed to put everyone ahead of you. It's good for the community for you to give, give, give until you can't give anymore. You're at the center of the ecosystem and your exhaustion means the system is working as it should.

"You're taught to be respectful, even though you're being disrespected," Denise Brown, 66, told me. "You're being taught to continue to go along and keep going and just sit in a corner and pray. And it'll eventually work its way out, but you're never taught while you're going through it to take care of yourself, to make sure you take care of your emotional and mental state because sometimes it can be overwhelming."

Other Gardeners noted that the pressures to be everything to everybody came from birth and didn't let up.

"My mama's a Black woman. My grandma, Big Mama, they're Black women," Latorsha Peake, 44, told me. "I know nobody ever said, 'Hey, just sit down, take a load off. It'll be okay.' You gotta get these kids together, you gotta clean this house. You gotta take care of your husband. You gotta be sexy in the bedroom. I really am in the space of giving people permission to do what it is that they need. It's not even about being selfish. This is just life."

But I did spot a shift. As I moved through the generations, a theme started to emerge. Conversations went from "I am the rock that society rests upon" to "Wait a damn minute, I matter too."

Rogena Burrus, 75, grew up as one of ten kids in South Central Los Angeles. For years, she watched as her mother took care of the kids, the grandkids, and anyone else who rolled through her house. On top of that, the house was always "spick and span."

Burrus spent years trying to convince her mother that she deserved some time to tend to herself, with her pleas falling on deaf ears. But Burrus realized that she inherited her mother's ways. "If I do not have something to do, taking up my day, I feel this sense of guilt that I'm not being productive," she lamented. "My day is always filled. And at the end of the day, all I can say is, *Lord, thank you for my bed.* But to just say I'm gonna stay in bed all day? I finally did it this year, maybe a month ago."

How did it feel? I asked. *Did you like it?*

"No," she said quickly. "I wasn't sleeping. I asked myself, So what am I watching on TV? While I'm in bed, maybe I can fold up clothes. Maybe I could get all this makeup off my dresser and put these things in place."

She heard herself talking herself out of a mental health day and laughed. "I'm always busy."

But now she recognizes how her daughter, now in her thirties with three kids, moves differently than she did as a young mother.

"She steps over their mess," Burrus said, laughing. "She's a nurse. She comes home from work and she tries to just sit down and lay down and she can nap. I can't even nap."

As we continue talking, Burrus pulls out a calendar and makes a note. "I'm writing it down. I should plan a me day. Once a month. At the end of the month."

I can't tell you how wide I smiled as her pen glided over the paper.

To shift out of the supreme caretaker role is scary. Won't it all collapse if I pull back and reserve more of me for me?

I'll be honest—it might. At least temporarily.

But a life that depends on your exhaustion to function is not a life worth preserving in its current form.

If you're still feeling some hesitation to shift some areas of your life, understand that your role as a helper and a nurturer is valuable. Your ability to care for the people you love and the responsibility on your shoulders is admirable. It's a skill, a gift that many wish they had. We should wear this as the badge of honor that it is.

My only nudge is to make sure you are *also* on that list of people you care for—at the top.

That's what this book is about: claiming what's rightfully ours and shifting the generations to come. This book isn't *Bloom How You Can*, it's *Bloom How You Must*.

Inside these pages we're crafting a new self-care legacy, a love letter to the generation of women who came before, who took what they had to create moments of rest, and a promise to us, the women standing on their shoulders.

Coming Home to Our Bodies

PHYSICAL WELLNESS

Are we feeling safe and at home in our bodies? Are we looking to escape from our bodies? Are we trying to numb what's coming up in our bodies? The art of coming home to your body, yes, it's an art. It takes time, it takes finesse, it takes intention and creativity and practice, but ultimately it is your birthright to feel at home in your body.

—Lyvonne Briggs, 40, pastor and author

EXPLORING THE ROOTS

IN 2015, SOUTH CAROLINA activists met and decided the Confederate flag—aloft on statehouse grounds since 1961—had to go. Bree Newsome, a 30-year-old filmmaker at the time, volunteered to snatch it down.

"You come against me with hatred and oppression and violence," Newsome bellowed from the top of the pole.[1] "I come against you in the name of God. This flag comes down today."

A year later, she spoke at a local university where I covered her speech for a client.[2] "A supervisor came over and directed the two officers at the bottom to tase me. Now, being attached to a metal pole, that could have electrocuted me. At that point, James [Tyson, a white ally] grabbed the pole and said, 'If you electrocute her, you'll have to electrocute me too.' And then they backed away."

When I heard Newsome tell her story, that detail—that she might be dead had a white man not intervened—stayed with me. Whose body gets protected? Who gets seen as precious and valuable? Why was the possibility of harm fine for Newsome but not for Tyson?

We all know the answer.

In every decade since 1619, Black women's bodies have been scrutinized, abused, endangered, judged, broken. It is nothing new to offer us up as a sacrifice for the "greater good" or to punish us for being out of order, as Newsome was when she scaled that pole.

Historically, Black women's bodies have been jobsites. Wherever we are, labor is also. We have been expected to be of service to others, day and night, inside and outside the home, to our own detriment. Our bodies were meant to be at work, regardless of how we feel or our desire to comply. As a result of that generational reality, now we often exist on autopilot. We don't notice the tension in our jaw or the dull ache in our lower back. We yawn but simply pour ourselves another cup of coffee and keep going. We struggle to keep our eyes open, but we do the dishes anyway. We may realize it's been a few weeks since we've had a good night's rest but do little to nothing to change it.

Our bodies are our most familiar companions, yet their needs and optimal functioning remain a mystery for far too many of us. How can we live a life that feels light and joyful and satisfying if we aren't in tune with our bodies, the vessel that gets us there?

In every event I host, my goal is for the Black women in my midst to feel good. Exuberant, even. We have enough spaces that are filled with doubt, sadness, and uncertainty. We need to pursue those spaces where pleasure is paramount. To hit that goal during the pandemic, I launched a five-stop wellness series I dubbed the Make Room Tour. Our penultimate gathering was a two-hour session on pleasure. Not just confined to the bedroom, but the type of pleasure that radiates in our skin and shows on our face. We were there to learn our bodies, express our desires, and pursue the good.

The guiding question for that session was, *Do you know what feels good to your body?* Do you feel capable of recognizing your body's signals that you are tired, hungry, overwhelmed? Do you know what to do to soothe your body? To bring it comfort?

For most of us on that call, the answer was no. There was a fundamental disconnect between what our bodies are telling us and what we do to meet these needs. How likely is it that your body is screaming out for attention? Mine was. I want to dedicate this chapter to us settling down long enough to listen to her and hear what she needs to tell us.

WHO TAUGHT YOU TO TAKE CARE OF YOUR BODY?

WHEN I WAS 5 years old and in first grade, my mom sat me down with an encyclopedia, gave me a pen and paper, and told me to read the section on "sexual reproduction." My assignment was to write a short report for her.

I don't know what sparked this idea—maybe she was watching the news and a report on sex education spurred her to teach me about the birds and the bees *right then*. Whatever her reasoning, I was already an avid reader and writer so I set about sounding out the terms in front of me. Fallopian tubes? Vas deferens? Seminal vesicles?

Marilyn, what is this?!

As far as my young mind could comprehend, sex was about fitting Ken and Barbie parts together. Little tadpoles and eggs were in there somewhere. After that, a baby would grow and come out of the mother.

Later that day, I gave my mother the paper, a few short sentences I hastily scribbled. In my cloudy memories, she read it and nodded her head in approval. That was the end of that.

That was my entry to the "sex talk"—very clinical and matter-of-fact.

It wasn't perfect but it was at least medically accurate. Later in elementary school, when I would hear classmates talking about "the stork" or some other euphemism for how babies are made, I would stride up to them with a "Well, actually" and lay all those rumors to rest. I was a third-grade sex educator, doing the Lord's work!

Outside of that early book report, I can't recall many explicit lessons on what it meant to care for my body. There were small sprinkles here and there. For example, my mother refused to have my ears pierced as a baby (a common cultural practice) and instead took me when I was 11, waiting until after I had asked, offering my first lesson in consent. *Nobody should do anything to your body you don't want them to,* she would say.

Outside of these small whispers, I learned that *taking care of your physical body is one of those things you get around to when you have time.* Other obligations—work, family, community—take precedence. I remember my family spending time together reading and eating. I remember vacations. I remember my dad working late and my mother studying for hours to pass her nursing exam. I don't remember anyone prioritizing sleep or setting a schedule for regular exercise. In my family, our physical well-being was more of a hum in the background than the focus of our days.

You may look back at your upbringing and struggle to find many examples of folks feeling good in their bodies or even being able to prioritize some type of physical care. Your memories may instead be filled with folks trying to get by or immersing themselves in the care and keeping of their family. Whatever your example, this is the perfect time to examine what your body needs and how to get it.

WHO TAUGHT YOU HOW TO TAKE CARE OF YOUR BODY?

- Did you receive any commentary about your body by adults in your family? How did they shape how you see your body today?
- Were you encouraged to exercise and move your body as a child?
- When it came to the sex talk, do you recall any conversations your caregivers had with you about pleasure?

- Were you able to talk about your natural bodily functions (like menstruation) or was it more hush-hush?
- Were you able to rest as a matter of household policy, or was rest something that was discouraged in your home?

LET IT GO

GEORGIA-BASED MASSAGE THERAPIST and self-care advocate Ursula Foster, 55, has been working to release the tension from Black women's bodies for more than a decade. The job, she told me, is getting harder.

"My work in massage is no longer enough," Foster said. "I've gone from giving sixty-minute massages to two- to three-hour sessions that consist of trauma work with sound, movement, and other modalities. It's difficult trying to get people to not wait till they are just completely on E before they book with me."

Foster owns a massage practice and retreat space in Stone Mountain, built intentionally to give her clients individual attention and let them know: *Sis, there is no rush here.* "I have clients that come in with their hair on fire and they're like, hurry up and get to it. It makes me go extra slow. I know it annoys some people, but I can't match that energy. If I match your energy, we're not gonna get anything done. So I slow down so you can slow down."

I love having women like Foster in my orbit because they remind me to stop rushing. Listen to my body and connect with her.

"That mind and body connection is real," she said. "I had a client recently where our session was almost three hours. We did massage, but we also stretched, we did yoga, we did meditation, we did this amazing twenty-minute womb affirmation. We did a yoni steam. We went through the whole gamut of her needs. And all she did when she came to me was she was like, *My hips are really tight*. That's all she said to me. But what I heard was, your hips are tight, but what are you holding in your body?"

I'm willing to bet that changed the direct trajectory of her day, her week, her month, I told Foster.

"The body is a very, very smart machine," she replied. "And once you tap intuitively into the systems of the body, it will do what it wants you to do and what it needs you to do without force."

Living as a Black woman through periods of upheaval is hard on the body. Full stop. In the midst of going about our daily lives—making headway in our career, raising beautiful children, nurturing strong relationships—we must also recover from the consistent onslaught of ways this society tells us we're too much and not enough at the same damn time.

Some of us find that healing through movement. From yoga to dance to hiking, moving our bodies allows stress to pass through. In *Burnout*, authors Emily and Amelia Nagoski educate us on the "stress cycle," the body's internal response to stressors in our lives. Stress isn't the villain we think it is, they write. It's getting *stuck* in the stress cycle that's the problem.

Stress is inevitable. We are constantly getting hit with problems we'd rather not have—a flat tire on the way to work, an argument with our spouse, a distressing news headline. Our problem is not that these stressors exist, but that we don't complete the stress cycle (*perceived threat—stress response—return to safety*). When we remain in that heightened physiological state for too long, our bodies start to go a little haywire—blood pressure rises, the immune system takes a hit, your stomach is upset more often than it's not, and so on. We think of stress as a mental phenomenon, but our bodies get hit as well. It's all interconnected.

The key to completing the stress cycle is to send your body the message that the threat is gone and you are safe. The quickest way to do that? Intentional movement.[3]

It doesn't matter if it's a five-mile run or a leisurely walk around the neighborhood. It could be tai chi. A Zumba class. Stretching on the floor of your living room. Whatever it is, your body will get the message that things are going to be okay. The Nagoskis recommend building in some type of physical activity to your daily life: "You experience stress most days so you should complete the stress response cycle most days too."

Like it does to many of Foster's clients, stress makes me tense. My whole body goes tight and my husband regularly has to spend time pushing my shoulders down away from my ears. My stomach clenches and my head starts to pound. It's an uncomfortable state to live in, yet my instinct is not to treat my body gingerly. It's to keep pushing through, like stepping on the gas when your engine is smoking.

It took me years to move my body when I felt stressed, instead of gritting my teeth and ignoring it. I will call up a friend and arrange to go for a walk. I'll drop down on my living room rug and do a few not-quite-yoga poses until I feel my body soften.

For some of us, though, it will take more than a ten-minute bike ride to soothe your body—and that's okay. "If you've spent a lot of years—your whole life, maybe—holding on to your worry or anger, you've probably got a whole lot of accumulated stress response cycles spinning their engines, waiting for their turn, so it's going to take a while before you get through the backlog," the Nagoskis write. "All you need to do is recognize that you feel incrementally better than you felt before you started."

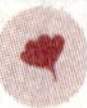

WHEN I GOT my first invitation to a yoga class, I imagined it would just be a lot of stretching. Maybe I'd sweat a bit, gain some flexibility, and leave feeling like a new woman.

I had no idea I'd be crying on the mat.

My first in-person yoga class was led by Dawn Rivers, owner of Daybreak Yoga studio in Ohio. It wasn't even a full class, just a small introduction to the practice as part of her Self-Care Sunday series.

At the end of the short practice, we moved into child's pose, a simple position that requires you to kneel on the floor, lean forward, and place your butt over your heels, stretching your arms out in front of you on your mat.

That pose requires an element of surrender, to let your body weight down on the ground, to connect with your breath as you release what troubles you.

Maybe it was something about sitting in community with other women, in my own space, on my own mat, that broke something open in me. Maybe it was residual stress I was carrying in my body that I wasn't in a space to recognize or heal. Maybe it was the feeling of safety. Maybe it was a sorely overdue pause in an overwhelming season. As Rivers instructed us to rise and do our final stretch, I felt the tears in the corner of my eyes: *What just happened?*

As best I can tell, I unlocked something simply by moving my body, a first for me. *This yoga is powerful.*

At its core, yoga is about stillness, breath, and spirit. Its primary function (as I've experienced it) is to help you get back to you. Or as yoga instructor and body positive advocate Jessamyn Stanley would tell you, "It's finding within life's shittiest moments the same flexibility, strength, grounding energy, and core awareness that you find in extended hand-to-toe pose or headstand."[4]

It was this grounding energy I was searching for when I tapped yoga instructor Saisha Baskerville to lead members of the Suite in a virtual session one month when the community was feeling particularly anxious. I wanted us to get together and breathe it out, and I knew Baskerville, with her inclusive approach to yoga, would be able to help all of us have a good time. The 31-year-old former high school math teacher turned yoga instructor came to the practice for the sake of her students, noticing that the calming nature might do a world of good in her classroom. But more than just an outlet for her students' stress and anxiety, it gave her the space necessary to address her deepening bout of teacher burnout. "There are years where you start [the school year] in September and are burned out by October," she told me.

But as a thicker woman, she struggled to do traditional poses, with her thighs and belly getting in the way of the streamlined stances. She looked for guidance from instructors and they looked at her sheepishly. *It can't be that hard to modify these poses for bigger girls,* she thought. She took it on herself to do what Black women do—create the resources they need. Thick Thigh Yoga was born.

"I was raised by a generation of people that were taught to take up as little space as possible to be hidden," Baskerville shared. "That you are gonna have to work twice as hard to get half as much. [Yoga tells me] I'm worthy of the moment to slow down, the mental clarity, the peace. We feel like we're not worthy of peace because we have to work so hard. We got all these bills and things like that. And while that's true, you're not going to get anywhere near as far as if you were well taken care of."

Her practice is about freeing women from the stress that lives deep within their bodies. "Imagine being able to sit down all of your stress or at least most of it," she offered. "Imagine being able to sit down your generational trauma. Imagine being able to sit down your financial stress, your physical aches and pains, your emotional baggage, your relationship stress, your family life. It would change your life, right? If you can put them down on the mat, if you can breathe it out, you can live so much longer and clearer and happier and healthier."

IN 2019 PATRICIA ANN CAMERON founded Blackpackers, a group dedicated to addressing the gap in representation in outdoor sports and leisure activities. Her Colorado-based organization partners with companies to donate gear and other materials to give Black families a head start exploring the outdoors without having to invest lots of cash in expensive equipment.

Her goal was to get more of us on the trails, ski slopes, and campgrounds and shift our historical perception of nature. "'Cause a lot of times it was work and/or how we fed our families," Cameron told NPR. "So it's not like we didn't go outside. It's just that sometimes outdoors was necessary to live, and that changes your relationship with the outdoors."[5]

Indeed, growing up as the descendants of enslaved people and farmers and sharecroppers shifts the way we engage with nature. Nature was a job, not an adventure. And even if we did want to explore the outdoors and revel in its splendor, it would do us good to remember the nasty realities of Jim Crow—until the 1950s, national and local parks were segregated, and public pools were off-limits as a rule of law. Due to decades of redlining and discriminatory city planning, communities of color are less likely to live within walking distance of parks, paths, and green spaces. And once we get there, we may not feel comfortable enough to stay. It takes a concentrated effort to enjoy the outdoors, which is why so many of us who do brave their excursions in nature choose to do so only within groups.

That effort is why I have never been an outdoorsy girl. Not as a child, not as a teen, and definitely not as an adult. I prefer cozy Saturdays on the couch, perhaps watching a nature documentary, but not actually experiencing nature myself. But thanks to a local hiking group, Black Women Explore (BWE), I'm now a Midwesterner who hikes in January. Willingly. Happily.

Thanks to one of those cozy Saturdays on the couch, I had been scrolling Instagram and saw a group of women I knew, smiling and lightly sweaty at the end of a group hike in the local Metroparks. After catching their big happy smiles for a few more hikes, I eventually commented: "How do I join?"

Five minutes later I had a link to the BWE Facebook group. Three days later I was on my first communal hike.

My friend Kimberly Young, cofounder of the group along with her good friend Bronlynn Thurman, gathered all eight of us in the parking lot and took a deep breath.

"Okay y'all," she said, her face emoting something I couldn't place. "How about we open up this hike with our intentions? What do you hope to get out of this time together?"

We went around and shared our hopes:

To let go of work stress.

To get clarity after a long week.

To jump-start some type of fitness routine and make it stick.

When it was my turn, I answered honestly: "To find community and get my blood pumping."

We nodded in agreement and set about on our three-mile hike. We huffed and puffed our way up rocky hills and slippery trails. We stopped to take pictures of flowers and beehives. We laughed. We sang a bit. We got lost. We laughed some more. We found our way back. Eventually we made it to our starting spot and posed for a group selfie in the parking lot, sweaty and happy. And my intention came true. I got my blood pumping and made several real friends from our treks.

When I talked to Young later about my first hike, she shared that she needed it as much as we did.

"I was having a horrible day leading up to it," she admitted. "I wanted to cancel. But Bronlynn probably would've strangled me if I did. So we went around and we did the intentions and I felt so much better because I was on the verge of tears. I can't even remember what happened, but I just knew that my soul was not right. And we went on the hike and afterward I felt so much better."

That communal time—being with our sisters in the midst of the trees—set us straight in more ways than one. We clocked three miles on that hike, taking about an hour to meander through the park. I average less than a mile when I go on walks by myself. What's that saying: "If you want to go far, go together"?

Nature is the perfect environment to let it all out, whether sweating up a mountain or running along the shore of your favorite body of water. Breathe and let it go whenever and however you can. Your body will thank you.

SWEET DREAMS

NOBODY WAS SLEEPING well in the aftermath of George Floyd's murder.

For the entire week after his last moments became public, I couldn't take a deep breath. Shallow breathing was all I had. My focus was gone. I'd open my computer and rapidly get lost in my own thoughts. And then at night, when I was trying to get my body to relax and let me drift off to sleep, sleep wouldn't come.

A quick survey of my friends let me know I wasn't alone. This felt like Trayvon Martin, Mike Brown, Sandra Bland all over again. *When would enough be enough?* We were walking through cement, our emotions big and unruly as we alternated between rage and utter disbelief. Our emotional reserves were already low after mourning the high-profile murders of Kentucky EMT Breonna Taylor and jogger Ahmaud Arbery in the months prior. Coupled with the emotions from a once-in-a-lifetime global pandemic, the hits just kept coming.

As the creator of The Self Care Suite, a wellness community for self-proclaimed "exhausted Black women trying to become well-rested," my job is creating restful spaces for us to lay down our troubles.

It was time to get to work.

I turned to my friend and yoga instructor Dawn Rivers to cofacilitate a free evening gathering I dubbed a "Decompression Session." I promised attendees: "We're gonna breathe, we're gonna journal, we're gonna let it out, and then we're gonna rest."

We needed each other.

Within a few days, we had women from all over the country gathered on Zoom to decompress in those precious moments before bedtime. We talked about how heavy we felt. How much anxiety had been stirred up. We journaled while listening to Erykah Badu and Sade. Then Dawn led us in a breathing exercise that left us all in awe.

Imagine thirty Black women, safe and comfortable in their own homes, coming together to exhale their worries and inhale strength from the group.

Inhale, exhale, inhale, exhale.

As I opened my eyes and let my eyes dart across the screen, I could see participants wiping tears away. We needed that release. *I* needed that release. A moment to breathe together, to let our breaths (virtually) connect and unfurl our collective tension.

It was magical.

We started hosting these sessions monthly, and I always left feeling lighter and ready for sleep. Attendees would report back in the morning, sharing screenshots from their sleep trackers to document how hard they slept. What a balm during an incredibly stormy time.

A few months after the first Decompression Session I got an email from a community member in South Africa who used the framework to host a session with her friends. "It has become increasingly necessary to have an online community to support each other in self-care," Masebe wrote.

All throughout the diaspora we were hurting and healing simultaneously.

When I developed the Decompression Sessions to help women in The Self Care Suite rest better, I was moving off pure instinct.

I don't have a degree in biochemistry. I wasn't aware of the delicate mechanisms required for a peaceful slumber. But I did know a little something from listening to hundreds of Black women: Daily stress prevented them from being able to wind down, relax their minds and bodies long enough to fall asleep and stay asleep, allowing them to feel refreshed in the morning.

For me, when my world feels heavy and the problems are coming at me faster than I can find solutions, sleeping well is often the first thing to go. I was desperate for a solution myself.

That led to an experiment. What would make it possible to go from frazzled and overwhelmed in the evenings to eager and ready for a restorative pause in our day? We could anticipate bedtime in the same way we anticipate a spa day, clearing room in our schedule and getting excited about the prospect of some pampering. Instead, for most of us, sleep is what our body forces us to do when we've truly had enough. We just kind of . . . shut down.

First, let's consider all the restoration that occurs when your body shuts down for the night. As Dr. Matthew Walker describes in his bestselling book, *Why We Sleep*: "There does not seem to be one major organ within the body or process within the brain that isn't optimally enhanced by sleep and detrimentally impaired when we don't get enough. . . . Sleep is the single most effective thing we can do to reset our brain and body health each day."[6]

Our nightly slumber acts as a housekeeper for the entire body, organizing, scrubbing, and categorizing all the remnants of the day.

Our brains go to work, deleting old memories that are no longer useful (what outfit your boss had on today, for example) and codifying new, important information (like what time your flight leaves in the morning). Our hearts receive a protective boost as well, with growth hormone being released to protect the lining of your blood vessels. Your body's fight-or-flight response is deactivated through calming signals your brain delivers to the body during NREM sleep to say: *It's all clear here.*

Without a proper night's sleep, your immune system takes a dive. Your reproductive hormones dip and make it more likely you will have irregular periods. Hell, sleep deprivation wrecks your actual DNA.

"It's easier to say what sleep doesn't affect than what it does," said Dr. Angela Holliday-Bell, author of *Sleeping on the Job*. "Sleep gives your body and your brain the time and energy that it needs to restore and replenish itself so that you can function optimally your next day."

Think of it this way: If I told you there was a single pill that would strengthen your immune system, regulate your hormones, provide greater mental clarity, and ultimately assist with your digestion and metabolism, you would sign up quickly for a thirty-day supply.

The good news is that "prescription" is already available to us through better sleep. So it's perhaps maddening—but not surprising—to learn that Black women get less restorative sleep per night than other racial groups, with higher rates of insomnia and short sleep periods.[7]

"Learning to rest was definitely not in my nature by any means," Dr. Holliday-Bell told me. "I grew up seeing my mom *hustle* and she still does, right? Sleep was never that important for us. We honestly didn't even really have real bedtime routines. It was all about working hard enough to get a good job to make money because we didn't grow up with that."

It wasn't until she went to medical school that she began to see the late nights and early mornings of training were turning her into someone she didn't like. She then inhaled all the medical data she could on sleep and volunteered at the sleep clinic to get a better sense of how she could help people, particularly Black people, get a better night's rest. The main way she shifts the culture? Leading by example.

"I wear a lot of hats, but one thing that I'm gonna do is sleep for nine hours at night," she said. "I don't know what else is happening, but during those nine hours, I'm asleep. Everything else has to fall into place around that."

Dr. Holliday-Bell's insistence that her rest is paramount moved me. If a doctor, wife, mother, and business owner could actively work to prioritize her sleep, then perhaps there's more room than we think to get better rest.

Lauren Wilson, 35, loved her work in higher education. When she was chaperoning a trip with her students, heading from their home base of Arkansas to Georgia, she didn't want to let her fatigue get the best of her. She did what she would normally do—she turned to caffeine.

That morning, she had a quadruple venti pumpkin spice latte. She followed that up with a Starbucks triple shot espresso. A little while later she gulped down a 5-hour Energy drink. All total, she had about 1,000 mg of caffeine coursing through her system.

At a rest stop, she got out of the van and noticed she felt funny. Next thing she knew, she was having a seizure and bit through her tongue.

Doctors ruled it a caffeine overdose.

Reflecting on that time, Wilson said she wasn't aware of how much coffee was her crutch to get through the day. "One thing that is normal is that I often wake up and I'm still tired. But I feel it especially when I've either been working really hard on things or when I'm anxious about something. I don't know what that means, but to me it's kind of a norm to be tired."

Wilson has a new job these days. But she's also completing her doctorate along with caring for her teenage daughter, stacking responsibilities like Jenga blocks. She already feels the pressure building, she told me, so she showed me her new calendar and to-do list, where there's a section dedicated to her self-care activities along with her homework assignments.

"I just have to find a way to do both," she said, shrugging. "That's very much a Black woman answer. You know, make a way outta no way. Find a way to make it happen. But when you don't have a choice, you don't have a choice. You just make it do what it do."

Let's make room for the possibility that, like Wilson, properly gauging our fatigue can be damn near impossible. Heavy eyelids and constant yawning don't necessarily mean it's time to get horizontal. What difference does "tired" make when you've spent most of your life watching people be tired and showing up anyway?

Anchoring your days around your sleep routine may feel like a luxury—and for you, maybe it is. But consider the cost of continuously missing out on the sleep you deserve. Insisting we can "get by" on six or fewer hours of sleep per night might be less of a biological reality and more of a mental crutch to make us feel better about sleepwalking through our days.

In one study, researchers measured the cognitive ability of two groups—those who were intoxicated at the legal limit and those who had been awake for nineteen hours.[8] Can you guess where this is going? Those who were merely "sleepy" performed just as miserably as those who were legally drunk, with a crash in their performance beginning to show as early as fifteen hours awake.

You know what you can "get by" on, now let's consider what we need to go through life at the optimum level.

Our ancestors kept a grueling schedule—up before dawn, working under the hot sun to particularly backbreaking labor. Research suggests that four hours of sleep was the norm. We can surmise that chronic sleep deprivation was the goal, to ensure that no one could have the mental clarity and physical capacity to do more than just survive the day ahead. And once they did manage to lay their heads down at night, that sleep was neither comfortable nor peaceful. The enslaved had such meager living conditions, cold and drafty with not much in the way of comfort. Add in the threat of violence (sexual or otherwise) and there is no way a good night's rest was possible. Imagine the impact that had on their entire life, and their children and grandchildren . . . all the way down to you.

Again, I insist: Our sleep deficit is deeper than the sleepiness you may experience on a regular basis. This is about the physical rest that has been systematically denied decade after decade after decade.

My maternal great-great-grandmother was a woman named Addie Barrett, born under the Georgia sun in 1866. She had twelve children in fifteen years and moved all across the American South, raising kids in Alabama and Georgia before heading north to Ohio.

I don't even have to know anything else to know that a well-rested Black woman, she was not.

Think back to *your* great-great-grandmother, a woman more than likely born in the 1800s. What do you think her sleep looked like? When she woke in the morning, did her bones ache? Did her mind feel clear? Was she able to greet the day with a smile? More than likely, she was perpetually sleep deprived, wringing the most out of each day and doing the best she could in a mental and physical fog.

Draw a line from your great-great-grandmother to you and let the urgency of the matter become clear. You deserve all the rest that is owed to your bloodline. You deserve to feel mentally clear, physically grounded, and spiritually full after a good night's sleep.

I want us to remember that we're human. We have the same needs as anybody else. Even when we didn't receive or weren't allowed to experience the space to rest, we have always deserved it. Let's claim this for all the women in our bloodline who deserved it as well.

For me, the hardest part of recognizing I need to prioritize my sleep is actually getting in bed on time. I regularly move through the day telling myself, "I'm going to go to bed early tonight," only to hit 11 p.m. and I am still awake, scrolling on my phone or watching TV.

I needed a better way forward, which is why I created the Decompression Method as a new bedtime routine. I recognized that I *did* have bedtime habits (what else would you call going upstairs and scrolling on my phone?). My routine just didn't have any structure and wasn't designed to move me gently toward slumber.

I needed something I could turn to and rely on to get me to sleep consistently and so do you.

You, dear reader, are carrying more than you realize. Not just today's problems, but those from years past that never quite settled in your spirit. The key to releasing what's troublesome is recognizing the weight of it all. We need consistent spaces to release, and I can't think of a better, more consistently available ritual than whenever you lay your head down to rest.

LET'S DECOMPRESS

THE DECOMPRESSION METHOD has three components. Each is designed to target one part of your wind-down routine—mind, body, and spirit.

First, *the Rubdown*. Start with a warm bath or shower. Dim the lights. Light a candle. The goal here is to signal to your body that you are ready for a slower pace. Make a playlist of your favorite songs. Once you emerge, rub yourself down with a lightly scented body butter, taking the time to feel your body, relax under your own touch. Sip some herbal tea, perhaps chamomile or lavender, to give yourself additional nourishment.

Next, *the Release*. Our brains can be an awfully cluttered place, with thoughts racing and emotions running high. Too often, we carry the day with us to bed and then wonder why we toss and turn.

When I'm struggling with something heavy that threatens to interfere with my sleep, I ask, "Who can hold this issue while I rest?" as my therapist taught me to do. It became the foundational question of the Decompression Method. Sometimes the answer is God. Sometimes it's a best friend. Sometimes it's the promise of an upcoming therapy session. The point is to think of yourself not as a solitary soul moving through the universe, but as part of a collective. I recognized that I tend to carry everything I'm feeling by myself (the whole reason I was even *in* therapy), and when she gave me permission to set everything down . . . I felt so free.

That's why the second segment of the Decompression Method is to journal and unravel those complicated thoughts that bounce around our brain during the busiest parts of the day. Often, we toss and turn because we are still grasping our concerns, clasping them to our chest like a favorite stuffed animal. Putting our inner world onto paper can help us begin to heal from those consistent, uncomfortable thoughts that stay with us, often the residue of a challenging or traumatic event. Or it's simply a process to get those mundane thoughts (*What's for dinner tomorrow? There's still a leak in the downstairs faucet. I need to get the kids new shoes . . .*) out of our head and onto paper so we can stop carrying them around.

This is where the journaling comes in. We are often told that we *should* journal but not *how* to journal. Ten questions, shared at the beginning of our Decompression Sessions, offer a solid starting point for most of us.

BEDTIME JOURNALING PROMPTS

- What has been the heaviest part of my day?
- What has been the lightest part of my day?
- What do I need to put down before I can rest well?
- What's one thing I can put on my schedule tomorrow to add some brightness to my day?
- Who can hold the biggest dilemma I'm currently facing so I can rest?
- What am I looking forward to this week that will give me a big sigh of relief?

- What is the biggest lesson I am resisting this week?
- What does an ideal day look like for me?
- Who or what can I turn to for comfort and support?
- What is the biggest lesson this week has taught me?

Once we have journaled, it is written. We will trust that our journal can hold it while we rest.

Finally, the third step of the Decompression Method, the breathwork and meditation portion, *the Relaxation*. This segment does the integral work of calming your nervous system, allowing your body to shift from a heightened state to a more embodied state. We're focused only on the present moment, asking ourselves: *Where am I at this moment? What do I see? What's in my hands? Is my body tense?* All these questions zero in your focus on the present moment.

I always thought that meditation was something I'd be able to accomplish only *after* getting my cluttered brain under control. It wasn't until I read Los Angeles–based meditation teacher Light Watkins's *Bliss More* that I realized it was precisely *because* my brain felt so cluttered that I was an excellent candidate for the wonders of meditation.[9]

In his chapter on "All Thoughts Matter," Watkins suggests that we need a tool to help us shift our mindset and find greater contentment in our daily lives:

> Why might our minds feel uniquely busy? It's been suggested that of the tens of thousands of thoughts we supposedly have each day, as many as 90 percent of them are recycled from yesterday. . . . In other words, without some sort of intervention like meditation, the way you felt about your life

yesterday is probably how you're going to feel about it today, tomorrow and the next day.

Meditation is the key that unlocks our stubborn mental patterns, offering new ones the space to grow.

A common misconception on breathwork is that you must do it in a certain way, for a certain amount of time, for it to have any lasting impact. As a breathworker, I've found that even a single deep inhale/exhale is quite effective in bringing calm to the forefront of your mind.

If you can, aim for ten minutes of slow, intentional breathwork and meditation. If that seems like an eternity, try it anyway. You are likely the type to be living in a heightened state, flitting from task to task so consistently that ten minutes of just breathing sounds impossible or overwhelming or boring.

What could be more inviting than to sit with yourself? To stop your world from spinning for just a few minutes and focus on the woman sitting at the center of it—*you*.

It is one of the most loving and grounding acts you can do for yourself, which is why it is the last item of the Decompression Method. Of course, when we facilitated these virtual sessions, there were women who routinely fell asleep during the breathwork portion, only to appear in my inbox the next morning telling me how much they needed that rest. If you fall asleep during breathwork, that's more than okay. However you do it, you're doing it right.

Take a minute now to notice your breathing. Does your chest rise and fall when you inhale and exhale or does your stomach fill with air? Chest movement means you're taking shallow breaths. No wonder we feel stressed! Without that extra oxygen flow, our bodies are tense and less likely to let go of the stresses they encounter.

My favorite yoga teacher always reminds us to open our lungs and audibly exhale. *Ahhhhhhh*. Take a moment and try it. Allow yourself to *hear* the stress leaving your body through your breaths.

Let's try an exercise: Lie on your back with your arms at your side. Close your eyes and visualize your entire body sinking into the surface you're on. Put one hand on your stomach, the other on your chest. Take a long, deep breath through your nose. Does your chest move? If so, try it again so that you physically see your stomach fill with air and your chest remains relatively still. Inhale for three counts, hold it for three counts, and then exhale for three. Work your way up to eight seconds for each inhale-hold-exhale.

In an ideal world, you'd have an hour to dedicate to your bedtime routine every night. But we know we don't live in an ideal world, so being able to complete all these steps may be a challenge some nights. However, the goal is to try to think about bedtime as an appointment on our calendar rather than a mindless event that occurs night after night.

Try these simple breaths as a starting point:

Exhale the stress of today, inhale the joy of tomorrow.
Exhale the tension in your shoulders, inhale the softness of your core.
Exhale the troubles of the mind, inhale the peace of the spirit.
Exhale the uncertainty of this moment, inhale the beauty of the future.

EMBODYING YOUR SENSUAL SELF

WE ALL DESERVE the space to embody our sensuality as a full and vibrant part of our self-care. Our bodies are designed for pleasure, no matter their age, shape, or ability. We deserve to feel good as we move through this life. What would it feel like if a pleasure-centered life was our default?

I must pause here and remind us that *sensuality* is not the same as *sexuality.* Sensuality, as sexuality doula Ev'Yan Whitney describes it, is "the process of being connected to your body, your senses, and what makes you feel good."[10] Our sensuality is as nuanced and multifaceted as any other part of our humanity—we don't have to all fit into one narrow box of what it looks and feels like. The most important directive (and yes, it's a directive!) is to shape and define it for yourself.

Sensuality is the container where our sexuality lives.

It can feel daunting to press pause and examine our bodies from a sensual perspective. Motherhood, age, illness, stress can all disconnect us from the fact that our bodies are wonderfully made. Through no fault of our own, we end up divorced from the possibilities of pleasure. It's a delight to remember how good it feels to, well, feel good.

Because there's a little distance between who we are and perhaps the sensual beings we'd like to be, I asked several Gardeners to share their sensuality role models, those people who exude sensuality in a way they'd like to emulate. Some were excited to share their sensuality role models (Jill Scott came up a *lot*) while others had to sit back a moment and think.

Writer Taya Dunn Johnson, 47, had to pause. She admitted it wasn't until her forties that she truly began to understand the difference between sensuality and sexuality. When she was in her late thirties, Johnson's husband, the only partner she had ever known, died suddenly. Her world axis shifted. She had to embark on a journey to relearn herself, after twenty years with the same man. "I had to say, okay, unlike my high school boyfriend who became my husband, who obviously had seen my body through all the transitions—from teenagehood through having his child through motherhood—now I'm a new person."

The prospect of dating again forced her to commit to loving on herself in a new way. "I've talked about this with my therapist, like, how do I really embrace my body and be body confident beyond 'I look good.' I'm not trying to be skinny for anybody, but how do I really embrace my curves? How do I really start to exude my own self-love and turn that into sensuality? What do I need? I started lighting more candles, taking more baths, taking pictures of myself in the mirror, talking to the parts of my body that I wasn't crazy about. I think that I put forth a much more confident, sensual version of myself, even when presenting to other people."

Even though her journey had been kick-started through tragedy, she ultimately became her own sensuality role model. I wanted to hug Johnson through the screen by the time she finished.

When I say "a pleasure-centered life," it means to move through the world like what you want is available to you. It's not confined to sex, although sex is indeed part of the equation if you want it to be. But centering pleasure is much more expansive—it is a full-body experience where your desires stay on the main stage.

ASKING FOR WHAT YOU WANT

SHORTLY AFTER VIOLA DAVIS got the lead role in *How to Get Away with Murder*, she arrived on set ready for a day of filming. Executive producer Shonda Rhimes stopped by her trailer for a little chat.

Aside from learning lines and bringing her overall *Viola MF Davis* energy to scenes, Viola needed to fulfill one more task—come up with a list of things that she, as the lead of the show, needed to make her happy. The list, Shonda told her, will ensure that Viola has what she needs to bring her A game every day at work. "Listen, you've got to be taken care of. This show rests on your shoulders," Viola remembered being told.[11]

I would love to tell you that Viola got right on it and came up with a list of twenty things that would make her time on set more pleasing. But wouldn't you know—she didn't. Later she admitted to still battling feelings of unworthiness after growing up dirt poor in Rhode Island. Her husband prodded her to complete the task. "Ask for some Greek yogurt. Some sparkling water. A massage. Something!"

We don't work in Hollywood so people aren't always going to come to us and ask to see a list of what makes us happy. But those items on the list should be known to you if nobody else. Release the idea, as Viola Davis had to do, that you are unworthy. Your crown has already been bought and paid for, as James Baldwin said.

The most liberating thing you can do is declare your desires, without hesitation, without wavering. *This is what I want and what I deserve.*

But what if you're like Viola and you're battling a lifetime of believing that a pleasure-centered life is for other people, not for you? Embrace your past. Remind yourself that you're new to this.

That was then, but this is now. You have *always* deserved this. Now you're coming for everything you are owed.

The first step is to have a conversation with yourself. There's no one else involved at this stage. Answer this question: *What makes my body feel good?*

I took a minute to jot down thirty things that made my body feel good in a nonsexual way and challenged members of the Suite to do the same. Here's a snippet of my list:

Warm socks
Linen sprays
Warm sheets
Warm brownies fresh from the oven
Warm shower right after a workout (but not necessarily the workout itself!)
Deep stretches, particularly child's pose
Getting my hair washed and feeling someone massaging my scalp
Soft fabrics
Having a fresh pedicure
Sitting on the shore of a big body of water
The way magazines feel on my fingers when I flip through the pages

These are simple pleasures, so simple in fact that you might not even notice them if you don't take a moment to observe. If you can't come up with a list right now, spend time over the upcoming week being intentionally mindful. Did you enjoy it when your coworker brought in donuts from the specialty shop next door? Did you happily accept when your partner offered to rub your shoulders? Were you excited to light the new candles you bought on your last shopping trip?

Pay attention to the little moments that make your face light up. They might continue to slide past you but once you capture them, they're in your mind and in your consciousness, which means you can begin to incorporate more and more simple pleasures into your daily life.

When it comes to owning our desires, we may be more fluent in verbalizing what we *don't* want versus what we do. It feels similar, right? What we don't want is usually the flip side of our desire.

One pattern I've noticed from coaching women is when we're coming up with our desires, we're usually coming from a place of lack. It's rarely *I want more of this.* More often, it's *Please let me experience something different.*

Parenting coach Natasha Nelson always tells parents, "Misbehavior is communicating an unmet need." I remix her mantra to say, "A complaint is an unmet need."

We complain about being strong for too long. What we're really saying is: *I need more support.* We are tired of being unappreciated. We're really saying, *I would like recognition for how hard I work.* We're stressed from carrying too much. We're really saying, *I would like my load to feel lighter.*

Adopting this "speak your desires" framework took time to adjust to. I'm a complainer by nature. If something is not right, you're going to know about it. Quickly! I don't believe in holding my tongue when something is troubling or unnecessarily stressful. If something hurts, I'm going to say "Ouch!"

But I've learned that while complaining feels good, advocating for yourself feels better. You know the saying—what you focus on grows. Focusing on what you *do* want allows you to begin to think about how to meet your desires, without focusing on the obstacles and challenges to get there.

Every time you start a sentence with what you *don't* want, pause and consider what you desire to be true.

"I hate being so tired in the morning" becomes "I want to feel well-rested when I wake up."

"I don't want to feel so lonely all the time" becomes "I want to have more friends to talk to."

"I'm tired of having sex that doesn't feel good" becomes "I want my sexual experiences to be satisfying for me."

Once you have voiced what you want to be true, it's easier for you to call in the support you need to make it a reality. You can then focus on a more diligent bedtime routine or a doctor's appointment to request a sleep study. You can be more intentional about accepting friends' invitations to hang out. You can speak up with a partner about the kinds of sex you enjoy most.

It took a concentrated effort to stop myself mid-sentence, reframe my complaint into a desire, and proceed with the conversation. It was like learning a new language. The more you practice, the more fluent you will become.

The reason speaking your desires works so well is that it allows you to truly embody a pleasure-centered life and give yourself permission to receive the pleasures. It's you at your most authentic.

LET'S TALK ABOUT SEX

BEING PARTNERED WITH the same man for twenty years means he has seen every sexual version of myself: the lusty teenager ready to drop it low at a moment's notice; the tired young 20-something mom of two small children whose exhaustion battled her libido;

and now the 30-something who gave herself permission to explore her adult sexuality without shame or fear.

Now that I'm staring 40 in the face, I'm realizing more than ever that sex is play! More than a way to connect, it's supposed to be fun. Sex releases a chemical cocktail of all types of endorphins and feel-good hormones all throughout your body. It's restorative, whether solo or partnered!

We may be struggling to embrace our sexuality as the vehicle for joy that it is, due to societal shame, religious upbringing, or a mix of both. Lyvonne Briggs, pastor and author of *Sensual Faith*, found the key to embodying her sensuality *and* sexuality in the most unusual of places.

"Having gone to seminary and been introduced to Black liberation theology and womanism and theology, I was like, what they been telling us ain't the real deal," she told me. "Our sexuality is a sacred gift. I'm saying that God desires that we enjoy healthy consensual sexual pleasure."

Through critical reading of the Bible and biblical scholarship, Briggs discovered the Bible is more progressive on matters of pleasure and sex than we were previously taught. Healthy, consensual *premarital* sex is indeed on the menu in the Good Book, according to different groups of scholars engaging critically with the text.

Take the Song of Solomon. Pastor and scholar Jennifer Wright Knust dissects it as a book that "celebrates pleasure for pleasure's sake."[12]

"Whatever this sacred poem means, whenever it was written and whoever composed it, the Song refuses to limit human desire to marriage or even to the love between a man and a woman," Knust writes.

The Bible, she insists, has no single ethic on what sex is, who's allowed to have it, and what it was designed for. "If one book recommends polygamy, the next recommends celibacy. If one revels in erotic desire, the next warns that desire is evil, a source of nothing but trouble. If one assumes that women should be prophets, the next tells women to sit down and remain silent. If one assumes that children and property are the aim of human life, the next longs for the sex-free life of angels. And so on. The Bible does not offer a systematic set of teachings or a single sexual code, but it does reveal sometimes conflicting attempts on the part of people and groups to define sexual morality, and to do so in the name of God."

These insights brought Briggs to a new understanding that she carried into her congregations, unafraid to speak frankly on our physicality and desire.

"When I think of being the bearer of a clitoris . . . you mean to tell me that God gave me this organ that has one job, and I'm not allowed to indulge in it when I say so? It is a part of our spiritual DNA to orgasm and to climax."

Our commitment to a pleasure-centered life, Briggs believes, will save us when the world is determined to run us low. "First of all, [sex] boosts your immunity. It releases stress. You're a Black woman in a racist, sexist, misogynistic, misogynist capitalist society. You need to relieve stress."

There's a slew of reasons why we might not know how to integrate our sexual selves into our everyday life. If you come from a family with a history of teen pregnancy, sexual trauma, or rigid ideals about "proper" sexual relations, what does that do to your own completely normal and healthy sexual development? We may be carrying sexual shame that doesn't even belong to us. Briggs wants us to get free.

"My aim is to remind women that the shame might be there, the conditioning might be there, but you are able to speak back to that conditioning, that voice that's telling you, this is wrong, this is demonic, this is evil. No, it's not. This is my birthright."

That shame can keep us bound and unable to fully engage in the quest of a pleasure-centered life. It's time to release the shackles and lean into the fullness of our being.

Stand boldly in your truth: *I deserve pleasure and as long as I'm not hurting anyone to get it, it's mine.*

If your sex life feels fulfilling and you get what you're looking for from most sexual encounters, then I'm happy for you. But if you feel like there's something lacking and you'd like for sex to be a more vibrant part of your self-care rituals, let's expand our minds together.

There are no rules other than the ones you agree upon with the folks in your bed. It doesn't have to look a certain way, certainly not every single time. You don't have to follow the pattern of *initiation-foreplay-penetration-finish*. You can do whatever you'd like. *Foreplay-penetration-foreplay*. You can do *only* foreplay. (Even as the term *foreplay* suggests that it's something you do before the "actual sex," as if it can't stand all on its own. It absolutely can!)

There's room at the table for an expansion of what sex can and should look like for us. For most of us, there's a couple unspoken rules of sex we tend to carry into our sex lives: One, for heterosexual couples, most encounters are penis-centered. It's in every sex scene or porn video: Once the man orgasms or loses his erection, game over. And two, there's a myth that women are notoriously hard to bring to orgasm (even though we know, in most cases, this is not true, looking at orgasm rates of lesbian couples).

Hence the orgasm gap.

This gap—the disparity of orgasm rates between sexual partners—exists in most heterosexual couplings. Black women's orgasms lag behind their partners at every age, with 75–90 percent of their partners reaching orgasm while only 53–75 percent of Black women they're having sex with do.[13] What do we do about that?

First, let's remember that orgasms are not the end-all, be-all of sexual activity. For a lot of us, being too orgasm-focused can hinder our sexual experiences and limit what could be an expansive and exploratory event into something much more by the book. What would sex look like if it didn't end when someone orgasmed? What if we just decided to ride waves of pleasure until we got tired?

But if you find that you *do* want more orgasms, that's a worthwhile goal. Orgasming more often requires knowing your body and what will get you there. Our erogenous zones are there for exploration, and it may take hitting two or more at once—otherwise known as a blended orgasm—to get you where you want to go.

Sometimes those sensations are a surprise (the back of my knee, really?), but sometimes it's as straightforward as hitting the main erogenous zones and seeing what comes up. Do you prefer slow, deliberate touching? Fast strokes? Do you crave friction? Pressure? A light touch? A more aggressive hand?

Pleasure mapping is a tool that can help you discover which actions can get you to the Big O faster. Once you know what you like on the menu (*ahem*), it's easier to order and know you'll walk away satisfied. Take ten minutes now to consider how you like to experience pleasure. There's as many ways to experience pleasure as there are seconds in a day, but this is a simple starting point. If it's a yes, place a Y next to it. If you haven't yet experienced an activity but are curious, use a question mark. If it's a hard pass, mark it with an N. Have something you like but it's not listed? Drop it in one of the blank spaces below.

DEVELOPING A PLEASURE MAP

Kissing	Showering together	Receiving oral	Giving oral	Clitoral stimulation
Masturbation	Food play	Fingering	Vaginal penetration	Anal sex
Missionary	Biting	Sex toys (external)	Sex toys (internal)	Sensual massage
Nipple/ breast play	Body worship	Talking dirty	Eye contact	Mutual masturbation
Role play	Multipartner/ threesomes	Cuddling	G-spot stimulation	Choking
Spanking	Public locations	Teasing/ edging	Sex praise	Hair pulling

These activities are mostly for partnered sex so bringing more pleasure into your intimate spaces requires good communication. We need to bring our partners into the experience with us. Ideally, everyone involved cares about everyone else's pleasure. If not, stop there and get a partner who cares if you're having a good time.

Sex educator and researcher Emily Nagoski offers one question to guide your sexual interactions: *What is it you want when you have sex with a partner?* Your initial answer might be: *an orgasm, duh.* But truthfully you can have an orgasm on your own or with a gadget designed to get you there. A partner is often not necessary for a climax. So what is it about *partnered* sex that you're craving? For you, it might be closeness and connection. It might be stress relief. It might be the feeling of someone else taking care of you for a little while, a period where you are not in control. Push that to the front of your mind as you begin the conversation.

This, again, goes back to our conversation on focusing on what you *do* want versus what you don't. That premise works well in the bedroom when you're in a mutually satisfying, emotionally safe relationship. Speaking about what you enjoy ("Go slow") is easier to follow than "Not like that." I'm all about increasing the chances of getting what you want, in all ways, always. This is an opportunity to guide you toward what you're craving.

"I'd like to have a sexual experience with you where you take full control."

"I'd like to have sex in a different room of the house."

"I'd like to spend twenty minutes just cuddling and rubbing each other."

Ooh, but I don't really talk like that, you might be saying. *It's hard for me to verbalize what I'd like, even if I know what I like.*

For some of you who feel bolder when you're not face-to-face, this conversation may work better over text. If you are in a long-term relationship and you want to improve your sex life for the better, perhaps spending time pleasure mapping together would be a good way to educate your partner on a slew of likes and dislikes at the same time. Whatever your approach, figure out a way that you feel comfortable, take a deep breath, and dive in.

We may not often be fluent in speaking our desires, particularly in an intimate setting, but continuing to shrink in spaces that are designed for our pleasure only ensures that pleasure will elude us. Use your voice and find the pleasure you deserve.

BRINGING IT HOME

YOUR BODY IS an amalgamation of everyone who has come before you. I see you got your mama's eyes, your grandmother's slender fingers, your aunt's button nose. Generations of people came together and their union created you. Isn't that miraculous?

It's our duty to hone our relationship with our bodies and love them through trauma, through disappointment, through stress, and back again. Celebrate our bodies for all they do and all they give us. Recognize how they've carried us, again and again, through life's storms without so much as a thank-you.

Think back to the last time you had to tell yourself to breathe. The last time you had to tell your heart to beat. The last time we had to tell our stomachs to digest our food. Our bodies are intricately designed vessels worthy of our praise.

Our bodies are home to wondrous sensations and pleasures. They also hold our deepest wounds and alert us when our environment feels unsafe or harmful to our well-being. They are our lifelong companions. Their needs must matter to us. It's not a matter of *if* we meet them but *how*.

Attention must be paid when our bodies are communicating with us. Go too long without responding and that "check engine" light *will* come on, leading to more extensive and expensive remedies to get at the core of the problem. It's easier to love her and tend to her before calamity strikes.

"Home is not an address," Lyvonne Briggs reminds us. "Home is where you feel safe. And your body is aching to be your home. So that no matter where you go, you feel affirmed, nourished, and loved. But that can only happen when you decide to embrace all of who you are."

Welcome home.

TEND TO YOUR PHYSICAL WELLNESS

THESE ARE ALL baby steps to get you thinking about being present in your body and exploring the many different pleasure possibilities. Go on your own personal sensual adventure and become an expert at treating your body well:

SPEND MORE TIME NAKED

Sleep naked, eat naked, watch TV naked. Get comfortable with your body in its current form. Notice your soft spots, your freckles, your firmness. Say "thank you" as you give yourself a squeeze.

SLOW DOWN IN THE SHOWER

While I know most Black folk will shun me for this, there is something sensual about forgoing a washcloth or a loofah and doing a direct skin-on-skin soap up. You get to feel every inch of your skin, gliding over your soft parts. Remember—even self-touch releases the feel-good chemical oxytocin!

CREATE MOMENTS TO DISCONNECT

You can't be in tune with your body if there's never a quiet moment to hear her. Practice the ritual of silence fifteen minutes a day—no TV, no music, no chatter. Hear what your body is trying to tell you.

GRAB SOME EROTICA

Explore some erotic audio story apps or listen to some new sex and love podcasts to get your imagination purring.

UPGRADE YOUR TOYS

If you haven't purchased a sex toy in the past decade, still getting by with Ol' Faithful, it's a whole new world out here. Clit and G-spot stimulators alone have changed the game. Browse and read the reviews to see which ones you're most intrigued by.

FIND WHAT MOVES YOU

You don't have to commit to a seven-day-a-week exercise habit, but more days than not, you can make some type of feel-good body movement happen. Complete the stress cycle, beloved.

ENTICE THE SENSES

At the core of being sensual is engaging all your senses. Spend some time exploring what feels good via touch, sound, taste, sight, and smell. New perfume, luxurious sheets, a delicious dessert—fill your life with experiences that delight the senses.

TILLING THE SOIL: PHYSICAL WELLNESS JOURNALING QUESTIONS

- What form of movement feels authentically good to you?
- What is your relationship to pleasure? Do you feel you deserve it?
- How can you expand your sexual freedom? What activities might give you a chance to explore your sexuality with intention and care?
- What does it feel like to be in your body? Asked another way, if someone visited your body and made themselves at home, what would they notice? What would they be comforted by or alarmed by?
- What daily practice can you commit to in order to learn your body's signals and needs?

Our Friends, Ourselves

SOCIAL WELLNESS

My mom had this social club called At a Moment's Notice. They even had a little logo and T-shirts. At one point they had a newsletter. They would meet maybe once a month. They would hop houses and every time it was at our house, it was always such a joy. My mom would get these little sandwiches, and they would just sit around the table, drink wine, and talk. And they had an agenda for what they were going to talk about. It would never be anything formal—they would just talk about what was going on in their lives. They would reminisce because a lot of them had been friends since high school, since college—a few were her sorority sisters. Seeing that and being an observer of self-care through communal work? It resonated with me. As an adult now, I'm very big on cultivating my friendships, especially my friendship with women.

—Angelique Dyer, 32, novelist and video producer

EXPLORING THE ROOTS

ONE OF THE most enduring visions of Black girl friendship has been the bond between media titans Oprah Winfrey and Gayle King. The two met in 1976 while working for Baltimore's WJZ TV station—Oprah was 22, Gayle 21. A snowstorm made for a treacherous commute home, and Oprah offered her house for a sleepover to prevent Gayle from being stranded, a gesture that sparked their fifty-year friendship.

Ever since Oprah became a household name with the launch of her show in 1986, Gayle has been part of the ride, appearing on the show more than anyone other than Oprah herself. We've seen them travel the country together, bicker over each other's hair and fashion sense, and celebrate each other in ways big and small.

"The real truth of our bond is that this is someone who saw me and cared for the essence of who I am," Oprah told *People* magazine.[1] "She became my mother, my sister, my friend. She became all the things I never had. I never had a strong relationship with anyone in my family who I felt really cared for me, really loved me, who wanted to hear what was going on in my life. I never called my mother or father to tell them anything that was happening. Gayle served as my chosen family. The person who stood in the gap for me."

That level of friendship often has folks coming up to the duo, eager to share stories of "their Gayle" or "their Oprah."

The truth is that Black girl sisterhood has kept us upright. It is the hair salons, the sororities, the postchurch chitchat, the kitchen table storytelling, and more that gave us permission to be free and let our metaphoric hair down.

It is that *I see you* and *you see me* that lifts our spirits.

The late great Toni Morrison not only explored Black girl sisterhood in novels like *Sula* but she experienced it, cherished it, in her own life with relationships with other single mothers, who provided her with a safe space after her divorce in 1964. I've long adored the stories she'd tell about her network of friends, including Toni Cade Bambara and Sonia Sanchez, who would take turns standing in the gap and providing the support that would allow all their careers to flourish.

"I remember [Bambara] coming into my house with two bags of groceries," she told Junot Díaz.[2] "No one asked her. She didn't say she was coming. She just appeared. She set the groceries down and said, 'I'll take care of the children today. You go do what you have to do.' You didn't have to ask. . . . That intimacy, that instinct, knowing exactly what a sister needed before she could even articulate it, was so important."

May we all know the joy of having a friend show up in ways that bring healing and peace of mind.

In an interview with Public Books, poet and activist Nikki Giovanni reflected on the communal atmosphere witnessed over her lifetime. "In my day, we used to come together, whether it was at the church picnic or we were just going by somebody's house to sit down and have a beer with them," she told researcher Pyar Seth.[3] "Whatever it was, we found comfort in each other."

When I spoke with DC native Alecia Velma Jackson, 75, she echoed a certain wistfulness about the beauty of community. In the 1980s, she was part of a group of women at her daughter's daycare who dubbed themselves "The Mothers," taking a communal approach to parenthood. "We took care of each other's children,"

Jackson said simply. "We had events where we just did things by ourselves. We would go drive to Atlantic City or drive different places to the beaches and just have outlets for the women. Then we did things with just the children in us. And then we did things with the husbands. And then we did things with their entire families. That lasted for about ten years." That decade of support taught Jackson a valuable lesson in community—we need each other.

Black girl community has been the blueprint. Who else was going to organize the rallies, the protests, the push for a better future? Black women have gathered for centuries, launching social clubs, political organizations, and sororities. Connection wasn't always focused on the individual (*our* feelings, *our* needs), but we moved collectively in a mighty way to ensure that our race would, quite frankly, survive.

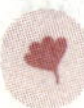

PREPANDEMIC, CIGNA RELEASED its Loneliness Index, where nearly four in ten respondents agreed with the statement, "I feel that I do not have close personal relationships with other people."[4] An updated 2021 study found that 68 percent of Black adults could be classified as lonely, a full ten percentage points higher than the loneliness rates among the total adult population (58 percent).[5] In 2023, the US Surgeon General released an advisory on the loneliness crisis, calling for individuals, organizations, and corporations "to make the same investments in addressing social connection that we have made in addressing tobacco use, obesity, and the addiction crisis."[6]

But why are we so lonely?

Sociologists have been studying our weakening social connections for decades, and one theory is the lack of "third places," a warm, accessible space to socialize outside of home and work.

In the past generations, membership at a home church might have fulfilled the bulk of our social lives. Between Bible study and time in the fellowship hall, we had a space where we could be among our people. For the nonreligious folks, amateur sporting leagues or social clubs might have held the same space on the weekly calendar. I grew up with a gang of relatives who spent evenings in bowling leagues and women's groups, spaces where shared hobbies and interests meant there was always someone around who "got you." They didn't have to wonder the next time they would see their friends and acquaintances.

But as the years went on, we've lost more of these third places than we can count. Between remote work, decreased membership in religious and civic organizations, and increasingly cozy at-home convenience, our social lives have taken a hit.

About a decade into working from home, I felt something was missing from my life. I was working and making a decent living, had two great kids, a nice house, reliable and funny friends. But it seemed like a huge effort to get out and be social. Where do I go to see folks?

I started hosting sister circles back in 2017. The first was in a basement office space owned by a friend, with about seven women in attendance, nibbling on mini sandwiches. We talked about what was happening in our lives, how we felt about our connections with friends, and what we hoped to accomplish moving forward. I had no idea what I was really doing, but I knew that spaces where we could be incredibly honest and raw about the realities of our lives were needed, a vital part of our well-being.

Our social connection is not simply an abstract concept, but the presence or absence of it shows in our physical and mental health. For Black women, the link between insufficient social and emotional support and depressive symptoms is glaring.[7] Research over the past twenty years has connected the dots for us—we're more likely to engage in unhealthy behaviors like smoking, poor self-care, and emotional suppression when we're feeling disconnected and unsupported from those in our social circles.[8]

In short, we're deeply unhappy when we're doing life alone. We need to find new ways of prioritizing connection, vulnerability, and community. Our well-being depends on it.

WHO TAUGHT YOU ABOUT FRIENDSHIP?

AS LOVELY AND warm as my mother is, I only have a few memories of her cultivating friendships. One is from my early childhood, when I was perhaps 7 years old. It's of vanilla ice cream.

My father had taken me and my younger two sisters to the mall. I don't remember why my mother wasn't there (maybe she was at work?), but during our shopping trip we ran into one of my mother's sorority sisters. Somehow the decision to buy ice cream came up and this woman went into her pocket and got all three of us a small cup of vanilla ice cream from Baskin-Robbins.

It was such a small thing—a sweet treat for some kids—but it imprinted on me, all these years later. My mother wasn't even present but her friend was so happy to see her children that she wanted to do something to make them smile.

As a child, I would sit and flip through photos of my mom's college years, admiring how happy she looked among her sorors, always matching in their pink and green. She had a small group that she hung with, and she would tell us stories about their shenanigans, with a bit of a laugh in her voice.

As the years went on, however, my mother's attention shifted to focus mostly on her family. She worked full-time most of my life, except for a few years during a career shift where she was toiling away in nursing school. On evenings and weekends, she'd be engaged with us, allowing her role as a mom to be her primary identity.

I took a lot of cues from my mother's life when I found myself unexpectedly pregnant at 20. As soon as I saw the two lines telling me I was indeed with child, I knew that as a Black woman raising a Black baby, there would be little room for error. As a young Black mom with very little money and a year left to go in college, there was even more pressure to "get it right." I threw myself into motherhood, vowing to be as present as humanly possible for my kids. While most of my friends were single and childless, they were all supportive. My best friend at the time voluntarily rearranged her class schedule so between her, my fiancé, and myself, we had round-the-clock childcare covered for the first year of my daughter's life. My friends would come over and play with her while I studied. They would regularly buy her picture books and clothes. They would keep her laughing when I brought her to our lunch dates.

For that first year, motherhood didn't change much about my social circle. It was my social circle that kept me afloat.

But after graduation, once we were no longer in the same proximity on a daily basis, those friendships weakened. My best friend moved to South Korea to pursue teaching. Others got different jobs, working second shifts and having less time to devote to our friendship. I had another baby and instead of leaning on my friends for support, I retreated, drowning slowly under the weight of my own and society's outsized expectations for mothers (especially young mothers).

Like my mother before me, I shifted my attention to the little people I lived with. Instead of shopping with my friends on the weekend, I was at dance recitals and Boy Scout meetings. I became a "room mom" and de facto field trip chaperone. I volunteered for story time and served on the PTA. I was there, in my kids' faces *all the time,* with little time remaining for myself.

I learned, however inadvertently, that *motherhood eclipses everything else, including friendships.*

When my children got older and I found more breathing room in my schedule, I doubled back on some of those prebaby friendships only to find them withered. It took tremendous effort to nourish those older connections and find new folks to replace the friendships that were too far gone.

I don't judge myself, my mother, or any woman who found her friendships gathering dust in the corner while tending to other areas of her life. Offer yourself grace if this is also your story.

We're all making do with the time and energy we have. All we can do now is course-correct and make our community a priority in the best way we know how.

WHO TAUGHT YOU ABOUT FRIENDSHIP?

- Who among your caregivers had friendships that modeled trust, vulnerability, and healthy communication to you?
- How often did your primary caregivers see their friends? Do you know what type of activities they did?
- What did your primary caregivers have to say about your early friendships? Were they encouraging and supportive or unenthusiastic?
- What did your early friendships teach you? Did you pressure yourself to "fit in"? Did you have to work hard to find "your people"?
- What societal messages have you absorbed about friendship between women? Between women and men?

FINDING YOUR (NEW) PEOPLE

THE BIGGEST PROBLEM I hear today is that once we hit adulthood, it's entirely too hard to make new friends. Once you hit your late twenties, you begin competing for time with people's preexisting obligations—their children, marriage, career, family, and existing friend groups. Truthfully, I don't know if it's hard to make new friends, or if it is hard to make new *good* friends.

It is not enough to simply find people who like us. We need to find people who are willing to do life with us. People who are intentional about maintaining our connection and willing to invest time and sometimes money into making it last long-term.

Connection coach Kat Vellos acknowledged that the stakes can be high when trying to make new friends, but let's relax a little. "One thing that helps is understanding that just based on pure logistics, it's not gonna work with every single person," she said. "And if we approach it as a little bit of an experiment, then it's a little bit easier to go in and discover, well, what does this friendship wanna be?"

The author of *We Should Get Together: The Secret to Cultivating Better Friendships,* Vellos reminds us that we aren't just collecting friends to say we have them—we're looking for real connection and support. "When we go in with this openness to really understand, who is this other person? What are they about? And they're understanding me and learning about me, it becomes like less pressure and a little bit more, 'I'm just learning what I feel like when I'm with them.'"

As we explore how to reach out to new people, we might hit the wall quickly. We do have those aforementioned priorities that aren't going anywhere. But the best way to get a friend is to *be* a friend, which means clearing space in your busy life for the friendships to flourish.

"Do a thought exercise on what your life would look like if you were busy with friendship," Vellos offered. "Because in either scenario you are busy, but the difference is what are you busy with? If you wanna be busy, be busy, but add friendship to your busy calendar, right? Or practice getting a little unbusy so it feels a little more spacious."

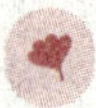

WHEN HABEEBAH GRIMES, 47, found herself at the helm of a major nonprofit, she struggled to find her footing among the demands of the job. The scrutiny, the demands of fixing problems that would take more than a generation to solve—all of it led Grimes to seek a community that could anchor her.

At that point, she had a few girlfriends she could call on, but she was looking to call in more. Specifically, she called on God to send her "the presence of divine feminine energy in the form of Black women."

Her prayers were answered, with Grimes meeting several women she wanted to develop relationships with. Some worked out better than others but every time she invited a Black woman out for coffee, lunch, a quick meeting, *something* good would result.

"The risk of seeking to spend time with a Black woman I admire was always worth it," she told me. "It always yielded a good conversation, thoughts of kindness and affirmation, upliftment, whether it was one conversation or the deeper relationships I have now through the village of women who are really consistently part of my life. I think of it as a divine kind of spiritual thing because I am a fairly anxious person and I can get stuck in my head and be sensitive."

Her process of building her community was a simple one. As she was out and about, if she met a woman she thought she vibed with, she would ask for some of her time to get to know her better.

What she was seeking in building her squad, she told me, was safety. "It gives me chills to say it, because I've never said this out loud or thought about it so deeply. But what these women have created for me is a sense of safety, and it's what I yearn to create for them. It's a place of reciprocity and mutual care, and that's been essential in these last several years that we've all lived through. I think it's going to be essential in the years ahead."

Every bit of our conversation felt like confirmation that new friendships are there for us to cultivate, however they originate. Sometimes hesitation on our part to lean in can get in the way. Will they like me? Will we click?

Were you nervous or unsure of how successful this was going to be? I asked Grimes.

She paused for a moment. "Our hearts are hungering for one another. I pray that we will all continue to take a risk and be vulnerable enough to seek out the community that we need because they need us too."

Let Grimes's successful pursuit of community and the abundance of her new circle inspire you to consider taking a risk. We are all seeking something, even if we don't know it yet.

While we're on the quest to find our people, I'd be remiss if I pretended that all friendships are easy to come by and that every friendship is always nourishing.

The real story is that relationships are often messy. We fall out. We hurt each other's feelings. We ignore signs that someone isn't able to provide what we need. We miss big moments. We get stuck in our own lives and forget to show up when it counts.

Those hurts stay with us as we set about trying to find our people. We may not be as open, or as hopeful, as when we were younger. We're guarded. Lowering our shield to access those vulnerable parts of ourselves takes time.

But that effort is still worth it to find those people who ride for you, who light up when you come into the room. Who will do the inconvenient when the situation calls for it. Who will tell you their secrets and hold yours close.

STRENGTH VERSUS VULNERABILITY

ASK ONE HUNDRED people to describe what they love about Black women and ninety-nine will probably give you something related to strength.

Ah, the Strong Black Woman. Known for the "S" on her chest, this woman is intimately familiar to me and most of the women in my circle. Perhaps you know her too. She looks like my grandmother, my hairstylist, my neighbor across the street.

She looks like me. She looks like you.

She is recognizable by her ability to show up, give wise counsel, and take care of business, over and over again, never fatiguing.

We are taught as Black women that we're problem solvers. We're dependable, we're reliable, we're wise. We have the wisdom, we care, we're nurturers, and we're incredibly strong. When you add all of those up, the messaging weighs us down like a life vest filled with concrete.

But the Strong Black Woman schema is not *just* about being resilient and capable—it has serious ramifications for our psyche. Psychologist Chanequa Walker-Barnes identified three distinct features of this mantle:[9]

Emotional strength is the central defining characteristic. "The StrongBlackWoman is supposed to be capable of enduring life's struggles without any sign she is under duress," Walker-Barnes writes. "She is expected to engage in constant impression management, maintaining control over her emotions at all times, especially those that indicate vulnerability, such as sadness, grief, helplessness, hurt, embarrassment, anxiety, or fear."

The second feature is *caregiving*, an occupation that is understood to only flow in one direction, from the Strong Black Woman outward to others. This is how so many Black women find themselves as the "reliable" one, the one people turn to for support without hesitation. That's what we're there for.

And finally, *independence* is the third feature, requiring that we handle life's toughest blows on our own, resisting help or support from even our loved ones.

Taking all of these features in totality, it's easy to see why it may be difficult for some Black women to develop nourishing friendships where they are able to be cared for as much as they care for others. This has been evident in my own work—in The Self Care Suite's community survey, 80 percent of respondents reported keeping to themselves when faced with a difficult situation versus turning toward their support network. Our socialization has denied us permission to pursue another role, one where we don't have to have all the answers, nor do we have to come to the rescue of others at the expense of ourselves. We'll handle it ourselves.

During a particularly rough season, where I was struggling to be a wife, grad student, an entrepreneur, and mother to two young kids simultaneously, I found myself on my white therapist's couch asking her to help me "learn how to manage everything better." Her response ("What if you didn't have to manage it by yourself?") knocked me for a loop. *What the hell is she talking about?* I thought to myself.

Unfortunately, the Strong Black Woman schema is self-reinforcing: We perceive that we have no support, so we endure everything alone, which makes it appear as though we don't *need* the support, so the cycle continues.[10]

Throughout the centuries, Black women have been required to be strong, to carry the weight of the community on our backs without complaint, without fail. As with most identities, it's a double-edged sword. Despite some of the psychological dangers, the Strong Black Woman identity has been a historical necessity—it's the armor that has allowed us to endure systemic racism and discrimination.[11]

As we sit with the realities of decades of socialization, we should ask ourselves: *Can we try on a new role? What would it look like to shed the armor and step into the fullness of our beings, ready to request and accept the support we so readily deserve?*

FRIENDSHIPS EXAMINED

OUR SOCIAL NETWORKS have three components—structure, function, and quality.[12] Think of structure as the *who*: the people who make up your social circle and their designated connections to you (family friend, neighbor, coworker). Function is the *what*: the value they add to your life (emotional reliability, financial support), while quality is found in *how you feel* about the connection.

You can have a highly populated social circle (*structure*), yet still feel unsupported (*function*) and lonely (*quality*). Conversely, you can have a smaller social circle and feel uplifted.

When my daughter was young, she peered over my shoulder as I was updating my Facebook profile. "Wow, you have over a thousand friends," she said, her eyes getting wide.

I immediately shook my head. "No, honey. These are just people I know. Well, kind of. Some of them I know, some of them are just . . . there." As I struggled to categorize the people whose lives fill my feed week after week, I wondered if we have watered down the label of "friend" and consequently, the relationship.

Picture This

YOUR SOCIAL NETWORK

Use the space below to map out your social networks. Work from your home outward, including people who live with you, your neighbors, friends, and family in your city, and so on, until you've included most of your closest contacts. Include the structure (who they are to you), function (what they provide), and quality (how their connection feels to you). See if you discover anything new about the levels of support you actually have versus the image you held in your mind.

Her question prompted a mass delete of tenuous connections. (A friend of a friend of a friend I've only spoken to once? *Delete.*) That interaction helped me clarify how I define friendship and be more intentional about cultivating and maintaining my community.

How did I get more than a thousand connections in the first place?

At each stage of my adult life, I turned to the internet to find my people and build community. When I was a young journalist trying to collect bylines, I found my people and built a network that would allow me to build a full-time career as a writer years later. When

I was a young mom, I started a blog to find other young moms to share how they were coping with this seismic life change. As a new business owner without access to coworkers, I joined entrepreneurship groups to help quell the loneliness.

Nourishing our digital connections is a new wrinkle to the human experience. For most of human history, we only had to maintain connections with folks we could reach out and touch. In a short amount of time, our networks have exponentially expanded, with social media allowing us—if we choose—to maintain connections with damn near anybody, from our best friend from kindergarten to our mom's favorite coworker.

There is a catch, though, now that our friendship networks are broader and more global. We can default to DMs and texts versus calendar invites and in-person plans. Technology allows us to phone it in, no pun intended.

Years ago, Brooklyn-born Naj Austin, 32, felt there had to be a better way to bring folks together than relying solely on a digital space. She launched Ethel's Club, a coworking and social space for people of color that baked in wellness from the start, with yoga and meditation classes available to members. The goal? To provide space for connection that mirrored her own life.

Austin gave me an example: On a recent Tuesday, she invited friends over to her brownstone to connect and unwind in a comfortable space. "My friends and I made dinner and we wrote poems to each other and laid on each other all night and that was for four hours. And that's like a classic day. Nothing about that night was special," she said, laughing.

Proximity is the point, Austin emphasized. Are we doing our friendships a disservice when we don't spend enough time in the same room, breathing the same air? Let's connect face-to-face, in real life, with the intention and focus we would give anyone we say is a priority.

"I would say that my friend groups are my lifeblood," Austin told me. "I only have friends who I'm obsessed with or I wouldn't call you a friend. And I take that very seriously because they're my community. They're the people who are going to help raise my children. They're the people who I move across the country for. They're the people who I would put in my house if they needed to be in my house. I think that because I'm a child of five, my mom's a child of nine, that I come from this large generous way of existing, from the space of abundance and how you share love and give love and receive love."

Austin's worldview inspired me to consider how much we rely on our digital connections to nourish us, in the absence of having proximate community we can reach out and touch. Social media allows us to easily create an abundance of "weak ties," those friend of a friend connections, which sociologists argue are good for our mental health and connection. But when we rely too heavily on those ties without *also* having a community of people to go deeper with, we can often miss out on some much-needed support.[13]

The goal is to have a diverse mix—good close friends that you can share life's challenges and celebrations with, acquaintances you can have fun with and learn more about yourself, and other weak ties to round out your daily interactions and infuse them with more joy. For now, let's focus on the people at the center of your circle, the people you would turn to in a crisis.

I call them your first responders.

WE NEED A FEW FIRST RESPONDERS

My bestie posted the following message for me as a birthday post a few years ago and I still tear up when I read it:

> I believe that God made Tara as an extension of His love for me, in human form. Our friendship has been one of the most rewarding relationships I've ever had and I'm so grateful.

Come on, somebody!

But the most beautiful thing about our friendship is that statements like this aren't rare. We regularly end our conversations with expressions of gratitude, an awareness for both of us that friendships where you can be your true, unguarded self are life-giving. We are happy we found each other.

She is my Oprah.

We've spent most of our decade-plus relationship on opposite sides of the country, with her home base in California and mine in Ohio. Our connection has flourished via our text messages and voice notes and FaceTime. We've been known to be carrying on several different conversations on several different platforms at once. Between family obligations and time zone differences, we learned to fit each other in to the open spaces of our lives, without much fuss.

When I called to ask her to speak at one of my events in Puerto Rico, she had no problem hopping on a bus, plane, and train to get there. When she told me she was having a graduation party to celebrate receiving her doctorate, I had my hotel booked before we got off the phone.

She is what I would call one of my "first responders," a friend who can easily swoop in and assess the situation when you need support.

First responders don't need to be brought up to speed on everything that's happened in the past three months. You don't have to spend a lot of time explaining what you need or where you are mentally. They are well equipped and available to be on the scene. Imagine you're having a really hard time, been struggling for months with work stress, family problems, and other obligations. Do you really feel comfortable unloading *all* of that on someone you haven't talked to since the seasons changed?

The beauty of having first responders is that they are not only there for you in tough times, but in the good as well. They can celebrate with you after a major accomplishment, give advice when you're struggling with a decision, or offer support when you're unsure of yourself.

It's imperative to have people walk through life with you.

My bestie is a person who knows what is going on with me and when. She often remembers the details of my life better than I can. I do not have to repeat stories and remind her of what I said last time we spoke. When I take a deep breath and start venting, she can gauge whether I need space or counsel.

When I coach women on finding more breathing room, it often means that we need to find them some first responders, which requires a level of vulnerability many Black women are unaccustomed to or have been punished for. Laying out our fears and anxieties doesn't always land well, especially when baring our souls to folks who don't know what to do or how to show up for us.

But it's still critical for us to be able to lay it bare.

Being able to say:

"I don't know what to do."

"I am tired. I have no more to give."

"I am overwhelmed. I need a minute to just be."

Knowing what we know about Black women's strength, you may not have a slew of living, breathing models of vulnerability. You may be infinitely more familiar with women fluent in keeping their deepest feelings close to their chest, quick to reassure "I'm fine" instead of the truth: *I'm barely hanging on.*

Let's rewind to 2007. My infant daughter had been crying for the past six hours, and as her shrill cries filled our cramped apartment, I was approaching my breaking point.

I was in my last semester of undergrad. I had gone to class earlier that day and was extra tired thanks to the sleep schedule a 3-month-old insists you keep. For some reason her father wasn't home yet to relieve me and let me get to my homework. I was standing in the middle of the living room/kitchen swaying softly back and forth, trying to get to the "happy place" in my mind. But her cries were too loud, too piercing. Any effort to visualize a warm breeze and a sandy beach quickly evaporated due to my baby girl's insistence for something I could not name. I had changed, burped, fed, rocked, swaddled, played, talked to her but nothing helped.

Later that night, after she finally calmed down and fussed herself to sleep, I took a long shower, put my face in the warm stream, and cried. *Why is this so hard?*

As time went on, I retreated to the shower more and more to let out my stress. It was the perfect escape. No one could hear me, and the water was so soothing. The shower gave me reassurance but also kept my secrets so no one had to know how much I was struggling in this new phase of motherhood. After I cried, I rinsed my soapy body and splashed my face with cold water to get rid of some of the redness around my eyes. I emerged from the bathroom with a temporary sense of relief.

A few months later, a friend confessed that she too cried in the shower, and I felt like we were members of a secret club. *See? I'm not alone,* I told myself. But after that moment of camaraderie passed, I asked her (and myself), "Why do you think we do that?"

"Well," she said carefully, "I don't want my son to hear me. I don't want to worry him, especially if there's nothing he can do about it."

And there it was. We hid our tears so we didn't bother our family. Not to show them that *hey, something is off balance here.*

In order to take "shower cry" off my to-do list, I had to start practicing real vulnerability—the art of being authentic about how you're feeling and dealing with the challenges life has handed you. As researcher Brené Brown tells it, I had to get comfortable with "uncertainty, risk, and emotional exposure."[14]

That meant expressing my feelings (sadness, anger, frustration, disappointment) right there, in the moment, instead of worrying about how it will sound or how others will view me.

I was moving from *self-silencing* to *self-advocacy,* an important leap if I were to do my part in receiving the care I deserved. I could no longer wear the mask of strength as my default.

Many of the women I interviewed found it difficult to drop their mask, having worn it most of their lives.

Natalyn Bradshaw, a multidisciplinary artist from Virginia, said that at 50, she is just now getting used to having a strong sisterhood to support her. "[In previous friendships] I was someone that would always show up for them. People will tell me as much, like, 'I know I can always come to you, Oh, you're so easy to talk to.' I took great pride in that. I still do. But what I understand now that I didn't understand then was that there was no one that was there for me."

Masking felt like the safest bet. "It has felt like I couldn't always fully be myself. But I always valued the relationships because it helped bolster my sense of self-worth at the time. So now the sisterhood that I have feels more like a sisterhood. And I say sisterhood—it's a very small circle. It's basically a dot," she told me, laughing. "I've got like two or three people that I know we've established a connection, that I know that I can go to them. I know that I can open up and I can be myself. I can maybe open my mouth and put my foot in it and I'm not gonna get ghosted."

Now with her chosen sisterhood, Bradshaw feels a shift in how she approaches emotional disclosure. "I feel like I'm back in school," she admitted. "This is something that I'm learning in real time. I have opened up, which is amazing. And I have been vulnerable. Right now I'm asking myself, What is safe? What is reasonable? Is this something that you can just hold for yourself or are you not sharing this because you feel shame or fear? I'm really learning to investigate and find the motivations behind whether I'm sharing or not."

"I've been able to share things with them that I'm like, *yo, I never thought I'd be able to tell anybody that,*" she said. "So as a recovering overachiever, a recovering perfectionist, that feels like an accomplishment."

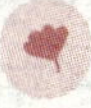

DURING THE SELF CARE SUITE'S mid-pandemic wellness tour, we hosted a small, intimate virtual session on friendship, drawing on members of the community who sought out connections with women who were also looking to make friends. A platonic speed-dating mixer, of sorts.

My good friend Valencia Joy was the cofacilitator. For the decade I've known her, she's been busy with the work of elevating our relationships and urging us to get close. She's author of her ode to friendship, *I Met a Guy . . . and Other Things You Can Only Discuss with Your SisterGirlfriends*. Her social wellness is top tier.

Our conversation got real vulnerable, real quick, as we shared how friendships have saved us in our hardest moments. Joy told us about the emotional minefield of attending her best friend's wedding, shortly after she discovered her soon-to-be ex-husband's affair.

"I excused myself to the restroom, but the minute I sat down at the counter, I started to cry," she shared. "Before I knew it, I laid my head on the counter and I wept. When I picked my head up, three of my friends were there. I never heard them come in; they never said a word. They sat there with me, rubbed my back. One of them wiped my nose. I haven't had my nose wiped since I was a baby! They sat with me until I was ready to go back."

That incident, and many others, cemented her vow to be open and share exactly how she was doing with her friends. "I love to tell my story, even the ugly parts, because I think isolation keeps us bound. We shouldn't act like whatever we're going through is so specific to us that nobody else has gone through it. I ain't the only one whose husband cheated. These things happen."

To be vulnerable requires that you lean in to your humanity, a reminder that your needs are not too much, too strong, or too heavy. Literally everything on Earth requires assistance to thrive. People, pets, machines, trees. There are no exceptions.

You, my good sis, are no exception.

PRACTICING VULNERABILITY

To be clear, I'm not suggesting that our lack of vulnerability is entirely our fault.

When we were babies, new to the world and learning how everything worked, we were loud about our needs. Our stomach rumbled? We'd cry. Uncomfortable gas? We'd holler. Need to get out of that wet diaper? We'd make some noise. As new souls brought earthside, we instinctively knew that we needed to make some noise to get assistance.

And somewhere along the way, that stopped.

Perhaps it was during childhood, when caregivers didn't rush to your side as quickly, instead admonishing you to "Stop making all that noise." Perhaps it was in your first friend group, when you struggled to be noticed and decided it was easier to play in the background. Perhaps it happened after you had dipped your toe into the pool of vulnerability only to find it shockingly cold and disheartening.

Whatever it was, it's good to acknowledge that we're not built to stuff our concerns down. We're social by nature and that innate desire means we need to lean on each other when times get hard and when times are sweet.

Think deeply about how you might respond to the following questions. Imagine it is a close friend, who is asking with genuine care, during a moment where you two have no place else to be and no rush to be done:

"How are you?"

"Do you need any help with that?"

"Are you okay?"

If those questions trigger a reflexive response that's somewhat dismissive, consider pausing to take a minute to check in with yourself. *Am I fine? What do I need help with? How is life going—truthfully?*

In conversations with the Gardeners, I found such beautiful connection when we could be real with each other. I would start each interview with an earnest "How are you doing today?" Some women were carrying a lot (a cancer diagnosis, the fresh loss of a parent or child) and it felt good, they told me, to admit they were struggling with it. Giving them the space to say so—to remove the Mask—was liberating for us both.

We lose so much when we put on the Mask.

The Mask is the protector. We can't get hurt if we keep people at arm's length.

The Mask wants us to appear strong and capable and engaging. The Mask does not like weakness and does not want anyone else to believe we have any weaknesses.

The Mask likes solitude. It craves distance. It does not want people to peek behind the curtain because *oh my God* you'll see us as we really are.

The Mask is the only reason a lot of us are able to get up and move through the world day after day. We are trembling under that Mask and very few people can take it off for us. For the most part, *we* have to decide when the Mask has to go. You wear the Mask because you don't want people to see you. But you forget that in wearing the Mask, you can't see yourself either.

RESIGNING AS THE STRONG FRIEND

As the oldest daughter and the oldest cousin, I've had this innate drive to make sure everybody around me was good. We're at birthday parties? I'm making sure there's enough cake to go around.

We're at the park? I'm making sure my sisters get a chance to play on the swings and go down the slide.

That same dynamic played out in my friend groups, especially when I was the first to become a mom. Someone has a headache? I have some Tylenol in my purse. You drank too much? I'm always the designated driver. Need to chat? Let me drop what I'm doing and give you a listening ear.

I had great friends, but I frequently kept them at arm's length, insisting that everything was fine. A sample conversation with me:

"Hey friend—how are you doing? How's [thing you mentioned two weeks ago that I made it a point to remember for our next conversation]? Oh really? That's great! I'm proud of you. You are amazing. Truly. Oh me? I'm fine."

[Narrator: She was most definitely not fine.]

For the most part, I do not carry any resentment toward the people I love. I enjoy making sure they're good. I like that they seek my counsel when they have a dilemma. I like being viewed as dependable and a safe space for those who need shelter.

The problem comes when the output and love only flow one way. When you're being sought as support but you don't feel comfortable seeking the same in return, partially due to your own fears and partially because no one thinks you need the same support you freely dole out.

The fear of being "too much" and the fear of losing my status as "the one who has it all together" are two burdens that go hand in hand with the Strong Friend burden I've worked very hard to release.

I had to swallow a deep truth: If I continued to pull away from people when they could potentially help me with situations that stress or overwhelm me, I would never have the support I so desperately craved.

Life, it turns out, is easier when you are working with a full crew. I enjoyed seeming well-adjusted and put together, but the truth is that I was no more stable or mature than any of my friends. We're stumbling through life together and I needed to practice letting my inner circle know that I am prone to tripping and stumbling myself.

I'd be willing to bet that most of the people in your life can and will support you once you make your needs known. For those who can't, forgive them. Release them from that position of expected support and sisterhood and let them be free to live their life. Holding on to anger about who showed up for you and when and how drains you. Turn your energy toward those who can show up wholeheartedly, even if it's only a handful of people. We don't need a thousand friends. Even one is a blessing.

WHERE EVERYBODY KNOWS YOUR NAME

SO FAR IN this chapter we've focused on the one-on-one relationships that are at the heart of our social circles. Practicing vulnerability, understanding what you're looking for, and prioritizing friendship are all important.

But our individual social connections are not the end-all, be-all to our social well-being. It is about *community*, that general sense of belonging and care among a group of folks that vibe with us. As we grapple with what it means to be in community with each other, we must find spaces where we fit. To belong is a human need, right up there with food, shelter, and love.

Sociologists suggest that having a regular "third place," outside of home and work, is key to good community building. Author Kat Vellos describes a third place as a space where "*it* belongs to you and you belong to *it*," a simple measurement for how community should feel.[15]

Where do you go outside of home and work? How long can you go (or have you gone) without walking into a space that feels like comfort, outside of your own home?

As we speak of the loneliness epidemic that has been brewing over the past few decades, part of the issue is the disappearance of regular, affirming community, feeling surrounded by a group of folks who celebrate your presence and who would notice your absence. And as technology continues to swallow more of our daily touchpoints with other humans, we'll have to be even more diligent about maintaining our connections.

I wouldn't be fair if I didn't acknowledge how the rise of digital connection has been a welcome development for huge subsets of society—disabled, introverted, or neurodivergent communities just to name a few. For some, digital connections are simply more comfortable, allowing them to share their true personality in a lower-stakes environment.

But we instinctively know (and research agrees) that the in-person connection touches our soul. Studies have shown that in the rock-paper-scissors hierarchy of connection, in-person outdoes digital but digital is better than nothing.[16] It's not a matter of *either-or* but ensuring vibrant third places are as much a part of our daily lives as our thriving digital connections.

Even as an introverted business owner who has worked from home for more than a decade, I've come to appreciate the value of a good third place, since my work and home lives commingle every single day in the same space. I've had to be incredibly intentional about the type of community I curate. If I'm not careful, I can go weeks at a time without having an in-person conversation with anyone other than my immediate family.

Years ago, I tearfully turned to my husband and told him I felt like I was suffocating socially. I had to make some changes in my life to build in more organic connection and curb my building loneliness.

I started hiking with the outdoors group Black Women Explore—our third place is the local parks system, where we alternate trails and enjoy the fresh air together. I joined a local young professionals' group where we met regularly to do service projects. I became a regular at a local coffee shop and struck up conversations with the owners, who believe in social good and also delicious gluten-free pastries.

I felt joy returning to me. I'd be invigorated when I got home, yapping a mile a minute to my husband about where I'd been and what I'd done. That type of energy in third places is why Vellos calls them "temples of belonging, self-expression, surprise, and connection."

WHAT DOES A THIRD PLACE LOOK LIKE? HOW TO FIND A THIRD (OR FOURTH OR FIFTH) PLACE

Clubs	Gyms	Digital communities
Service organizations	Churches	Coworking spaces
Hair salons	Libraries	Cafes/bodegas
Bookstores	Parks	Lounges

Sociologists define a third place as an actual location, within walkable distance of your home, where you can go to socialize and relax without the pressure to buy anything in exchange for your presence.

Unfortunately, thanks to car-centric urban planning, suburban sprawl, and unrelenting capitalism, it's hard to find a third place in an organic way. Outside of those who live in major metropolitan areas, most of us aren't going to be able to slip on our shoes and find a bustling, vibrant community gathering space within a few feet of our front door. And that's a shame but also not something we can fix short of moving, with the hunt for suitable third places front of mind.

Let's instead think about what is possible for us and how we can find and create spaces where we are able to let our hair down, without the responsibilities of home and the professionalism pressure of work. Instead of "third places" I call them "joy spaces," places that may or may not be proximate, but they soothe the soul all the same.

WHAT MAKES YOUR SHOULDERS DROP?

A good third place is a place that feels like *you*. If you can't be your authentic self there, it's a waste of time.

Start with those activities and hobbies that you like. Are you a creative, looking for a space to explore all those ideas swirling in your head? Do you need a place to get physical and bust a sweat? Or are you an intellectual, desiring a place to talk with those who get you? Consider what type of vibe you're looking for so you can know where to begin.

HOW MUCH CAN YOU INVEST?

A third place is ideally free, but a joy space might cost something, however small, to access. Notice I said "invest," not "spend." Some spaces, like a community center or library, may be free, while others, like a gym or café, require a minimal fee or purchase.

WHAT'S ALREADY AVAILABLE?

Before we start trying to create an ideal joy space, let's see what already exists. Consider the distance you're willing to travel to reach this destination. Make sure you factor in your other obligations, which likely will shorten the distance you're willing to consider. If you have to drive an hour to reach this joy space, you probably won't go there often.

Do a deep dive into this radius. What is available for you to make your own? Vellos asks participants in her workshops to get curious about the world around them, researching if there are under-the-radar places that could fit. Sometimes that research is as simple as living life and paying attention when opportunities cross your path. I was at home scrolling on Instagram when I discovered Black Women Explore. My husband approached me about a young professional organization he heard about at work. I joined a digital group for gluten-free foodies, which led me to frequenting the coffee shop with the delicious muffins and cookies. Being open and curious about what already exists can help you skip all the labor of having to create a joy space all on your own.

What if you try all this and you still feel you're coming up short? Your joy space may not be a place but a person. You may not have a brick and mortar location to retreat to, but perhaps you do have a couple friends who give you the same feeling a third place or a joy space might. Cultivate those relationships and wherever you are together, that's your joy space.

TEND TO YOUR SOCIAL WELLNESS

AS WE LOOK to nourish our social ties, understand that our social wellness can be the trickiest to ensure because it is not solely up to us—other people and their priorities will also have an impact on how strong and flourishing our friendships are. But that doesn't mean that we can't take ownership for our side of the equation:

ASSESS YOUR CAPACITY

While our social connection is exceedingly important, most of us have full and busy lives, which means we must figure out how much time we can dedicate to nurturing our friendships. Do weekly check-ins work? Monthly meetups? Most of us won't have time for daily connection, but as long as the connection is meaningful, it doesn't have to take place every day. The key here is to strike a balance—if it's too frequent you run the risk of overcommitting; too infrequent and you miss out on valuable support.

COMMIT TO YOUR FRIENDSHIPS

Are you complaining about how lonely you are but you've flaked on the last three sets of plans you've made with friends? It's tempting to cancel for any number of reasons—it's cold, you're tired, there's nowhere to park, you don't have anything cute to wear. But you'll be surprised how much your life improves when you make the commitment to be a woman of your word. As much as humanly possible, show up when you say you will show up.

GET ON THEIR CALENDAR

Life is too hectic and too busy for us to always arrange friendship meetups on the fly. We can do better by finding a regular time to meet, perhaps on a monthly or a quarterly basis. If you can't do that, make it a point to arrange the next meetup when you're leaving the current one. Spontaneity is great but having regular touchpoints with your friends allows you one less thing to think about.

PRACTICE SHOWING UP IMPERFECTLY

Sharing how you feel *after* you have sorted yourself out is not true vulnerability. (Shocker, I know.) As Black women, we tend to isolate when sad and reappear when we've got things under control again. If this is you, let's consider letting people in ever so slightly and see how things shift. You don't have to be perfect to be seen.

BE COMMUNITY MINDED

Adopting a community mindset means you view the world through a lens of collaboration and mutual benefit, leaning on the principle of interdependence. Your core belief is *We need each other to survive*. That means you need people and people need you. For some of us, this is easier to believe than it is for others, especially if we've seen people go it alone our whole lives, never witnessing true reciprocal relationships up close. Remember to lean in to your humanity, the very essence of which requires social connection and belonging.

EXPAND BEYOND YOUR PEERS

Intergenerational relationships provide opportunities that simply connecting with your peers doesn't. How can you connect with women who've walked your path before you? Much has been made about the disconnect between generations, but I've personally learned to lean in to those differences and appreciate the quirks that emerge when our generations collide.

PRACTICE DOING LIFE TOGETHER

Finding time to prioritize friendship doesn't have to be a complicated endeavor. It can be as simple as an invite to the things you already do as a matter of habit. Invite a friend to the laundromat or the grocery store. Instead of just going online to make a purchase, find a local store and make a trip to check it out. But more than that, make it a point to *be there*. Send a "just because" card when you know they've been having a tough time at work. Make it a point to ask about their kids' music recital or performance review at work. Be invested in the day-to-day and see how it comes back to you.

TILLING THE SOIL: SOCIAL WELLNESS JOURNALING QUESTIONS

- How many strong, reciprocal relationships do I have the bandwidth to nurture right now?
- What are some of my interests that can lead to a new connection with people who also share that interest?

- What gets in the way of building the relationships I desire (e.g., time constraints, compatible prospects)?
- Where do most of my close friends live relative to me? Is this sufficient?
- What is my love language and how can my friends show up in ways that feel loving and considerate to me?

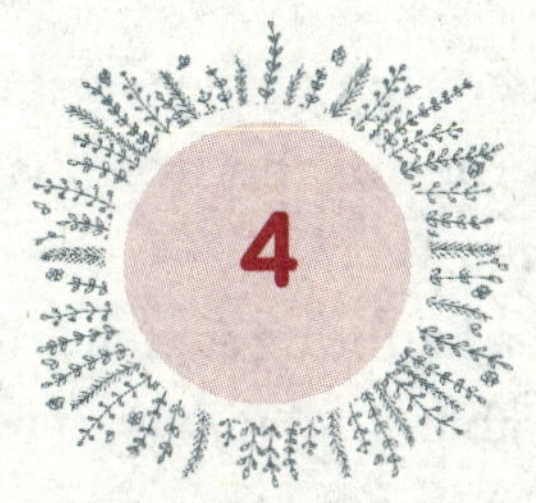

Carving Our Own Lanes

PROFESSIONAL WELLNESS

Don't stay where you're not celebrated. A check is never worth that. That lesson is hard because I still have to take care of my children. I still have to live life. I can't just quit my job because I've now cussed out my manager again because they were talking to me crazy. I have to do things differently and put plans into place so that I can obviously continue to live and support our lifestyles, but also be at peace. In my younger years, I wouldn't have done that. I definitely have stayed in positions where I was miserable or people were disrespectful. I knew I had to pay the bills and that's a hard lesson.

—Aneesha McGregor, 43, nonprofit executive

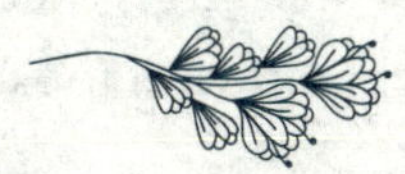

EXPLORING THE ROOTS

IN THE OCTOBER 2, 1918, edition of the *Greenville Daily News*, a slim article tucked in the corner of the front page bears the headline: *Negro Women to Be Put to Work.*[1]

The piece opens with a haunting sentence: "Regardless of whether they want to or have to, able-bodied Negro women who are not regularly employed are to be put to work, put in jail or fined heavily."

I first stumbled on this article when it was shared by Tricia Hersey, founder of The Nap Ministry, a global movement to persuade Black women and the world at large that "rest is resistance."

My curiosity led me down a rabbit hole to quickly discover that not only was this proposed ordinance real, but in 1918 several cities across the United States were passing similar measures specifically targeting Black women, demanding their labor.

The Greenville City Council drafted the ordinance after labor shortage complaints from white people. Black women were sitting at home, collecting checks from the government, they alleged, and they needed to return to their proper place—in the homes and fields of white families, doing the same backbreaking labor that they had been forced to endure for the previous three hundred years.

What's often lost in all this is that some Black women *were* at home receiving government checks—the marginal benefit of being married to servicemen who were off fighting in World War I. It was their right to be in the home, taking care of whoever needed tending to, even if that was only themselves. City council members were not wringing their hands over the labor participation of white military wives, whose labor was largely seen as voluntary if not outright discouraged. Black women who took this time to tend to their families were seen as criminals for refusing participation in the labor pool. Should the ordinance pass, they could be stopped on the street and asked to see their "labor identification card," proving they were gainfully employed and not, as their white counterparts were able to do, spending their days as they damn well pleased.

Similar struggles were taking place around the same time in Pine Bluff, Arkansas, where for the first time in their lives, monthly allotments from their husband's military service allowed some Black women the option to say no to low-wage work in the fields.[2] (We're talking $1 per *100 pounds* of picked cotton, equivalent to about $20 in today's dollars.) Furious that their perennial labor force had opted out, planters put pressure on local politicians and business leaders. The Pine Bluff Chamber of Commerce (who knew they wielded so much influence?) petitioned the US Secretary of War to grant them the power to arrest these Black women, citing their protest in violation of the nation's wartime "fight or work" mandate. Miraculously for the time period, the War Department sided against the planters, informing them that Black women would likely go back to the fields for better wages and working conditions.

The laws were popping up so fast that the NAACP issued a direct message to President Woodrow Wilson to issue a "prompt condemnation of efforts" to force Black women back into the workforce.[3]

These are just headlines from *one* year of Black women's lives. Of our mothers, grandmothers, and great-grandmothers.

A 1990 study tracked the leisure activities of Black women born in the early twentieth century and in the workforce during this time. Most spent their professional lives in domestic or agricultural work. Nearly all respondents either reported that they had no leisure time or they shared "leisure activities" that sounded suspiciously like . . . work.[4] Grocery shopping. Cleaning the house. Cooking.

No wonder we are at war with our professional lives.

As I talked to Gardeners of a certain age, they shared their "almost" careers. One wanted to be a television anchor; another wanted to be a dancer. More still expressed a desire for a bolder, more creative career but found themselves in administrative positions, work they did well for decades, despite their longing to follow a different path.

Those professional diversions were sometimes self-selected; others were signs of the times. For Gloria Clifton, 62, growing up in Pine Bluff meant that the vision for young Black girls' future was very narrow.

"When I read Michelle Obama's first book, *Becoming*, about halfway through, I put that book down and I thought to myself that she had something in her childhood I did not have," Clifton told me. "And that was people who supported her endeavors. Growing up in the town that I did, that was not something that many girls got. For wanting to be anything other than a nurse or an administrative assistant. If you wanted to do anything outside of that realm, it was always a pushback. And I just felt had I had the type of support that she talks about, how her parents supported her, how teachers supported her, how people at church supported her, then I think I might have done even greater things in my life if I had had that type of support."

Clifton went on to retire from the pharmaceutical industry at 54. *You are one of few women I've talked to who have actually retired*, I noted during our conversation.

"Well, I've been working since I was 9," she said, sharing how she would spend her summers working alongside her mother as they cleaned white folks' homes.

Oh, so you put in your time, I said, laughing.

She laughed with me. "I've done enough."

I've done enough.

Our professional careers span most of our lives. We may not traditionally think of careers as a space to be well, but we spend more time immersed in work than almost any other endeavor. It would do us well to consider how we move, professionally, and if there's any opportunity to shift into a higher space of well-being.

Gone are the days of having a single employer, working there for thirty years, and retiring with a nice pension. Now, the job market is oversaturated, job-hopping is touted as the best way to beat inflation, and retirement will be largely self-funded.[5] We have an opportunity to transform the way we think about work completely.

At its core, professional wellness is having your gifts and talents affirmed in a space where you are paid appropriately for your time and energy. But it is also about the space to not sacrifice your sanity and your well-being for the almighty dollar. It's about pursuing a financially successful life on your own terms—of all the facets of wellness in this book, professional wellness might be the most hard fought of them all. Our legacy in this space is fraught and comes with generations of sacrifice, pain, and restriction. Even in our fairy tales, like 2009's *Princess and the Frog,* we're working two jobs and facing discrimination because people can't see that we're human! Let's figure out how we can do this . . . better.

WHO TAUGHT YOU HOW TO BE A PROFESSIONAL?

THE MOST ENDURING memory I have from my mother is of work.

I absolutely remember the smiles and hugs. I loved being in the kitchen when I could smell her famous breakfast potatoes—only potatoes, onions, and salt—getting golden brown on the stove. I remember her "Good morning to you" wake-up greeting, sung to the tune of the "Happy Birthday" song.

But truthfully? When I think of my mother, I think of a woman who *always* had a job. Even when she got laid off or left a job for one reason or another, she seemed to get a new job before I could blink.

The summer before I left for college, my father got laid off. Then, crazy enough, my mother lost her job a few weeks later. With both parents unemployed, I immediately felt like I should delay college, at least a year, until things could stabilize. In a few short months, we would really begin to feel the pinch, with us possibly losing the house we had called home for the previous fifteen years. I couldn't possibly add college tuition on top of everything else.

When I told my parents I was prepared to delay college a year, they responded in tandem: *No, you're going now.*

The nursing industry being what it is, my mother found another full-time job relatively quickly. My dad's job search—he was in sales—was taking a little longer. So my mother picked up a second shift at a different facility to help keep the roof over our heads. This meant she would go to work at 8 a.m., put in a full day shift until 5 p.m., attempt to sleep from 6 to 10 p.m., only to be up in time to start her 11:00 p.m. to 7:00 a.m. shift.

I watched her run herself ragged. As a college student, I tried to do my part by maintaining my grades and getting additional scholarships, but seeing how hard my mother was running her body into the ground for the sake of her family will never ever leave me.

"We were behind in our mortgage payments and I didn't want to lose the house," she told me. "I didn't care about the consequences. So I just did what I had to do."

I did not realize until I interviewed her for this book that she maintained that schedule for *eight* years. Even after my father got back on his feet, relatively soon after she got hired at the second job, my mother continued that grueling pace for nearly a decade. Her second job allowed them to not only keep the house but contribute to three college tuitions and rising costs of living.

It was a hard conversation. I had to ask her if she thought it took a toll on her, health or otherwise. "Had I not been doing that, I would have had time and energy to focus on other things," she admitted. "Just having more me-time, to focus on myself so I can have meditation or mental health time. Spending so much time working two and three jobs like that, you tend to neglect yourself."

My mom told me she got her work ethic from my grandparents. My grandfather worked at Manchester Steel until his death, and my grandma remained employed with the City of Cleveland until her retirement. They never called off work. The pride in my mother's voice was evident.

"One day, my father's car wouldn't start," she told me. "It was a blizzard outside. I watched them walk to the corner, in the middle of the street, arm in arm to go to the bus station. *In a blizzard.* To go to work. I was only 5 or 6 years old. I will never forget it."

From watching her up close, I learned that *it is possible to do the impossible when you have a family to support.*

As I was coming into my own as a professional, I began to unconsciously pattern my own work ethic after hers, just as she watched her parents in the blizzard.

I worked relentlessly in college to set myself up for a promising journalism career. By the second semester of freshman year, I became editor-in-chief of the Black on-campus magazine, a title I held for the next three semesters. I was managing editor of the main (read: white) on-campus magazine, while writing for the LGBTQ magazine and holding a spot on the editorial board of the campus newspaper. I chaired the student chapter of the National Association of Black Journalists. I was also freelancing from my dorm room, nabbing hundreds of bylines with low-budget and no-budget online publications, making exactly zero dollars. (It pisses me off to think of how much I have written that is lost to the internet recycling bin forever.)

By the time my senior year arrived, however, so had my daughter. Determined to have a baby and not miss a beat, I completed all my work for fall semester by Halloween and had her three weeks later. I did not know at the time that Title IX protections would have given me extra time to complete assignments; alas, no one told me. With a throbbing C-section incision, I limped into class in early December for finals. My final semester I took Reporting Public Affairs, which meant I was supposed to cover city council meetings and be out in the streets writing stories. I strapped my daughter on my chest and went to work. (I got an A minus.)

Upon graduation, I got a job at a local nonprofit, where all went well until I found out, ten months into the gig, that I was pregnant with my second child.

It took a minute to get up the nerve to tell my boss—a middle-aged white woman—I was expecting. When I did, she looked concerned and sat back in her chair. Her first question? "Will you be returning to work after the baby?" I swear to you, dear reader—until that point, I truly didn't even know becoming a stay-at-home mom was an option!

In her world (and I suppose as a boss), it was a valid question. But it stunned me. Nearly sixteen years later I still remember how I eked out a confused "Um . . . yeah?"

In my lineage, motherhood only means you pick up *more* hours. Babies can't eat air.

After I got laid off from that nonprofit job three years later, I decided to start a consulting firm, in part because I've never wanted to be tethered to an organization but also due to the rising cost of childcare. I figured I could watch my kids (then 4 and 2) *and* build a blossoming business.

Sense a theme? Overworking was normal to me. I had no reason to think anything I was attempting was out of the ordinary. I had watched my mother do much more.

I got to work, building my client base. Before I knew it, I had five different clients, offering each of them twenty hours per week of my time. (You do the math.)

I would kid myself into thinking I wasn't working too hard because, hey, I was working from home. So what if I was working eighteen-hour days, six days a week? Who was I to complain? I had no boss. Nobody was making me.

Yet . . . there I was, overworked and underpaid, like so many generations before me. I knew there had to be more to my story than just putting my head down and grinding until I retired.

Or would I even get there?

A series of health hiccups took me to urgent care, where I sat across from a doctor who looked at me with real concern. After she gave me a directive to rest for a full weekend, I recognize that she might have saved my life.

I spent that weekend in bed, contemplating how I got here. I decided I had to make some changes, income be damned.

I let go of all but one of my consulting clients. I prepared myself to take the financial hit, but the gag was, I was so underpaid that losing four clients didn't matter all that much. I committed myself to therapy. I joined a gym. I tried to resuscitate some old friendships that I had neglected in pursuit of professional success. I turned to my young marriage, which was withering due to neglect from both ends.

I had to make big changes. And I did. This is also the period right before I launched The Self Care Suite, having seen how Black women need more than Instagram captions to help them heal. We need community. We need opportunities to hear each other think. We need an introduction to a new way of being, *especially* when it comes to our professional lives and how we tend to ourselves while we try to make ends meet.

In all the areas of our lives that require our intentionality, our careers sit front and center. In a capitalist society, we *must* find some way to earn a living, whether at a nine-to-five or if we're wearing the boss hat. Regardless of how you earn your coins, there's wellness to be found.

WHO TAUGHT YOU ABOUT PROFESSIONALISM?

- Did you grow up lower/middle/upper class? What would you say you are now?
- Did any of your primary caregivers enjoy their jobs or look forward to the workday? What do you remember about their careers?
- Were you encouraged to go to college and have a career according to *your* interests? Or were you put on a specific career path at an early age?
- Have you ever had a job where you were encouraged to bring your full self to your workplace—your style, your speech, your way of being?

DEFINING SUCCESS

BEYONCÉ HAS PRODUCED a lot of content for the last twenty-five years, and I've studied her 2013 *Life Is but a Dream* documentary relentlessly. It premiered around the time that I was beginning to feel some symptoms of burnout in my career, although I hadn't yet begun my investigation into what that actually meant.

At this phase of stardom, Beyoncé was working hard to revise her vision for her career, after blasting through with Destiny's Child and enjoying a solid ten-year run as a solo artist. In the documentary, she's figuring out her next move, wondering what success looks like for her.

"I don't want to have to sing about the same thing for ten more years," she said plainly. "You can't grow. I decided it was time for me to set up my future."

The decisions she made then—becoming her own manager, setting up Parkwood Entertainment, focusing on cohesive bodies of work versus radio singles—set the stage for the superstardom she enjoys now. The documentary forced me to rethink how I define success. When I began my consulting firm after getting laid off, my only goal was that I wanted to make the same salary working for myself that I did when I had an employer signing my checks. And I made it, in slightly over a year. But still, the "success" also brought insane working hours and too many consecutive "Nos" to girls' night out invitations. There had to be more to success than money. This was barely living.

I had to revise my definition. Money aside, what would make me feel like a success?

My new definition is simpler: *I want to rest more than I work.*

When it first occurred to me, I recognized that if I achieved it, I would likely be the first woman in my family to experience anything *close* to it. I'll admit—considering that context, it made me feel a bit lazy. My great-grandparents and those further back in my family tree did real physical labor most days of their lives. Running a farm, raising dozens of kids (both their own and those of the white families they worked for), picking cotton and rice and tobacco. And here I am making a goal of fewer hours sitting comfortably in front of my computer?

I had to sit with that discomfort and recognize the truth: Most of us aren't running farms nowadays, nor are we expected to live just like our foremothers did. Times have changed, thankfully, to a world where I can earn money using my gift of the written word. I'd like to think my great-grandmother would be proud of my work-life balance, not ashamed.

My goal of rest > work keeps me focused on what is truly important to me. I desire a life that is more than meetings and budgets and project calendars. I want to travel. I want to support my children in their endeavors. I want to experience time freedom. I want so many things that have nothing to do with how many hours I'm sitting at my computer, being "productive."

For me, it's liberating to stop counting pennies as I try to determine my measure of success. Because sometimes, despite your best efforts, you will suffer a defeat: you may get laid off, a new client might not work out the way you hoped, or a promising deal will fall through. It happens to the best of us, and tying our self-worth to our bottom line isn't healthy for us, mentally.

Whether you're in corporate America or calling your own shots as an entrepreneur (or you're doing both!), it's up to you to figure out what success looks like. If you don't know what you're striving for, how do you know if you're headed in the right direction?

Now, for those of you who fear taking money out of the equation, realize that your personal definition of success can include an income goal, but an income goal alone is an incomplete definition of success. Here's a few questions to help you brainstorm:

- What do you want your life to feel like on a random Tuesday?
- What experiences or behaviors do you want to be able to have? Think about charity, travel, and so on.
- What would you like your family to remember about you after you're gone?

Success is personal. It's perfectly fine if your version of success isn't about late nights grinding, but rather about being able to go to bed at nine. It's okay if you count yourself a success if you have the flexibility to attend your kids' recitals and games.

Wellness advocate Liz King, 72, grew up in a multigenerational home watching both her grandparents work jobs that were less about personal satisfaction and more about putting food on the table and a roof over their heads. Her grandfather was a Pullman porter, while her grandmother was a hotel washroom attendant.

"Their hard work, which I know was so often discriminatory, punishing, demeaning, and boring, gave me golden opportunities to experiment with my life and be free-spirited in new ways," she told me. "They allowed me to try things that they themselves had never tried before. They empowered me to take permission to fail, to be different, to adventure, and to be solidly unconventional."

Her version of success is honoring that gift.

"Doing the things I love most is my highest contribution to society, my legacy, and the best example I can set for anyone who cares to look at who I am," she continued. "Being true to my nature—recognizing and honoring it—is the most gratitude I can give to my parents and all of the ancestors who brought me here."

As women who have grown up with the knowledge that we can do so much more than our ancestors could, there often comes a point where we conflate *what we do* with *who we are*. But our professional lives are only a slice of who we are in totality. Achievement feels great but we are so much more than a title or a position in an office.

Social media has undoubtedly fueled a rise in this comparison trap. I've heard countless stories of influencers renting homes because they feel their spaces don't fit the "aesthetic" they're trying to portray. You can fall into a trap if you're looking over your shoulder at another person's life, trying to gauge your level of success by their standards. Keeping your eyes on your paper, as my therapist likes to say, is the best way to measure your own success.

Developing our model of success often requires a complete mindset shift. Our role models often had one goal in mind: *I need to be able to pay the bills.* It was survival, plain and simple. Anything over that was gravy. This means we can feel a bit rudderless when we are trying to envision our path.

In speaking with the Gardeners, it became clear: What we've seen isn't necessarily what we want to be.

North Carolina native Alisha Robertson, 35, knew she wanted something different, even if she had never seen it herself. "I always saw my mom and all the other women in my life working one and two jobs that they hated, that was often very physically strenuous on them," Robertson said. "It don't matter if you don't like the job, don't matter if the job is stressful, there was no talk of mental health and how all of that weighed on them. It was: *you work and you make it happen because you have no other choice.*"

With every iteration of her career, Robertson said, she's been burnt out and stressed trying to hold it all together. Once she had her daughter, she recognized that she wanted to model something different—for both her daughter *and* her mother.

"Now that [my mother's] retired, she told me she's been working since she was 12, 13, and has never taken a real vacation," Robertson told me. "So one of my goals is to be able to take her on a real vacation. 'Cause now she's worked all these years and she doesn't have any other life experiences to show for it, you know?"

THE POWER TO PRESS PAUSE

FOR YEARS, THE biggest event of The Self Care Suite was our annual retreat, Here We Grow. We would typically gather in the fall, somewhere between September and November, for an extended weekend of self-care, sisterhood, and exploration.

These events were mostly a one-woman show (me) in the early years, and the team would never grow larger than two. It's seven months of work to bring each event from idea to execution.

After the retreat, I'm spent and the only thing I want to do is rest.

That is how my sabbaticals began.

After the first retreat, I took two days off. I was riding high off the event and was still very much in workaholic mode. I was acting president and volunteer coordinator of Team Do Too Much.

After the second? I felt a little more freedom (and a little more run-down) so I took two weeks.

By the third and fourth, I planned to be out of office for a full month. It felt so good to step away that I stretched it to two months.

In 2019, our fifth year, we had just come back from a five-day excursion in Puerto Rico. It gave me clarity on exactly how much I had accomplished in my years of building the Suite. I gave myself time—in this case three months—to figure out what would be next.

I gave myself from mid-November until mid-February. I love that the holidays are tucked in there and I could be fully present with my family as we celebrated the end of a long year. My goal was to slow work *way, way, way* down and fill most of my waking hours with a to-do list focused on pleasure. It's tending to myself in ways that are difficult when the majority of my waking hours are about work. In previous years that has looked like:

- Getting a huge pile of books from the library (I love books and libraries in equal measure) and striving to read one each week.
- Spending extra time loving on my husband.
- Working on home renovation projects like my bedroom and home office makeovers.
- Pulling out my cookbook collection and making dishes that are usually too fussy to make during the average weeknight or trying to perfect some of my favorite family recipes.
- Assessing my wardrobe and personal grooming to see what needs to be adjusted.
- Catching up with friends to lay eyes on them and see how life has shifted since we last spoke.
- Sleeping as much as I can and lounging around the house in the softest, coziest clothes I own.

This, truthfully, is not much different from how I approach my day-to-day life. I'm a self-care coach and community leader and I take that shit seriously. I do my best to practice what I preach and that involves having ample time in my life to rest and do what I need to do to feel centered. I take mental health days as often as needed. I begin most mornings by writing a "comfort list," three or four items that I want to incorporate into my day to put a smile on my face.

But while I love my daily bits of ease, by the end of the year I'm craving something more substantial.

My sabbatical helps me get a broader picture of where I'm at in my life. It's my yearly time-out. I can take my time because I know there's no big project on the horizon that I need to be preparing for. I can let my mind wander. I can explore things that are important to me without feeling like they're getting crunched in the endless list of More Important Things.

How can I afford it? First, a few notes: My husband and I split the financial responsibilities of the house. Other than our mortgage, we don't have any debt. No credit card bills, and miraculously no student loans, which lowers our monthly expenses considerably. In the months leading up to the sabbatical, I cut back on my spending and take an extra project here or there to give me a cushion.

For members of The Self Care Suite, I let them know it's sabbatical time. I preschedule content so it doesn't go completely dormant, and I will drop in on a weekly basis to see how it's going. But I release myself from the pressure of being present for everyone else when I know my tank is empty. I show up when and where I can and the rest will fall where it may.

I wish every Black woman the opportunity to have an extended leave from work to *just be*. From the time we reach maturity, and for some of us even earlier, we're spending a good chunk of our lives either in somebody's office, dealing with office politics or some form of entrepreneurship.

What we need more than ever is a space to step back and catch a breather. This need is why Chicago native Reesheda Graham Washington founded Sweet Rest, a for-profit organization that funds flexible sabbaticals for Black women.

"We always think that making more money is what's gonna get us to the rest," Washington told me. "But honestly, you can think when you rest. You can be creative, you can be innovative, and you find your way into ways to make more revenue without killing yourself."

She started the organization with Kaitlin Rogers Perez, designating it as a for-profit organization to allow the flexibility to move as the spirit led, without getting caught in the slow pace of the nonprofit world. In the beginning, they approached sabbaticals in the traditional sense—you need a break from work, they got you. But they quickly realized the truth of Black women's lives was more complex.

"We were being too prescriptive in years one and two," Washington said. "We needed people to tell us what makes your shoulders relax, what makes your heart rate settle? What makes you thoughtful about your own way of being in the world? 'Cause that's what rest really does."

Their sabbaticals began to take unconventional forms. One recipient, resentful that her hectic work schedule prevented her from really connecting with her kids, used her sabbatical funds to take an extended staycation in their hometown of Chicago. Another used it to get Sisterlocks so she could release so much focus on whether her hair was "done" to her standards.

One beneficiary of the work, Halleemah Nash, used her sabbatical as a career break to figure out her next move after a decade working her way up the corporate ladder. Her Sweet Rest sabbatical allowed for fifty days of renewal, nearly seven weeks that Nash spent reading, meditating, and practicing yoga.

"I wanted to make sure that how I define rest was from sort of a decolonized perspective," Nash told me. "So I connected to Black women, I connected to Indigenous populations. I went to yoga initiatives in South Los Angeles that were in the Slauson and Crenshaw neighborhood. I wanted the idea of rest to still connect with my identity."

She came out of the sabbatical with clarity—she was going to launch her own business. But with that discovery was a commitment to making rest a permanent practice: "Rest can't just be something that you do when you are on vacation, rest can't just be something that you're doing when you're recovering from something."

For some of the Gardeners I spoke with, their sabbatical was merely a pause button in a busy life. For others, it shifted the entire trajectory of their lives, like Delaware native Stephanie Perry.

For her fortieth birthday, Perry took a weeklong trip to Brazil. While there she ran into a group of 20-something globetrotters on a quest to see as much of the world as possible. They opened her eyes to the possibility of life being more than clocking into an office.

"I wasn't on a journey to find myself," Perry told me from her hotel in Puerto Rico. "I wasn't even on a journey to restore or recover from burnout or anything like that. I wanted like one piece, one chunk, one year of my life where I could do whatever I wanted, be wherever I wanted for as long as I wanted to be there and not have my job be the boss of me. All I wanted to do was see all these places in the world that were my screen savers on my computer at work."

As a pharmacy technician at a hospital making $22 an hour, she was ready to try something different. Her goal was to start in Thailand, where she wanted to try authentic Thai food and witness the Loy Krathong festival, where more than half a million candlelit floats glide down the city's rivers and ponds, allowing people to make wishes for good fortune.

She set her plan in motion.

Over fifteen months, she saved the $14,000 she would need for travel expenses. She planned on visiting places where the United States dollar stretched further, where she could spend $500 a month on an Airbnb and have plenty left for food and sightseeing.

She quit her job. She surrendered her home back to the bank and sold most of her belongings so she didn't worry about storage while she was gone.

"I started working around 17 or 18," she said. "I'm probably gonna work until I'm 67. I just want a year while my body is still on my side. I wasn't asking for the world. Seventeen to 67. One year out of fifty. That's not a lot."

In September 2015, she left Delaware and landed in Thailand, a month ahead of the lantern festival. Over the following year, she visited twelve countries, spending months in Southeast Asia, South America, and Europe. All that adventure gave her a new vision for her life. "My career break introduced me to 'Agency Stephanie,' to the version of myself who feels I have control over my life. I am in charge of my life, and I have a say in how I live. Every single decision is totally different from what it would have been before."

Once she returned to the United States, she realized she wasn't ready to let go of her wanderlust. She quit her job three months later and began to make plans to become a "forever traveler," using housesitting gigs to see the world on her own accord.

So the plan went from one year to . . . indefinite? I asked her. *Was reentry to the United States really that jarring?*

Oh, but it *was*, she told me, almost shuddering in response. "Work is really the sun in our solar system," she said simply. "I didn't notice. I thought that was just how life was for everybody. I thought that was just life in the twentieth and twenty-first century. Going out there and seeing that it wasn't like that for other people? I didn't wanna come back to it. We really don't get to be whole people. And yeah, that sucks."

Perry began coaching women on taking a career break, guiding them through the process of obtaining visas, finding remote jobs, and even the hurdles of traveling with kids.

Women think it's the money holding them back, Perry told me, but really, it's the belief that they actually *deserve* to put themselves first.

"Black women only get praised out in the world, or even in our own families when we're exhausted," she mused. "When we're doing everything for everyone. Letting go of that means you're letting go of the approval of everyone in your life. Most of the time money can be figured out. But the real fear that pops up is, who am I if I'm not the *fill in the blank*? If I'm not *this job*, if I'm not *this superwoman*, if I'm not *this doer of everything for everyone*, then who am I? It's really scary to stand on that edge and know that you don't know yet. You haven't met her."

If you're reading this and thinking, *Well, this must be nice but it sure as hell won't work for me with the way my life is set up*, please know that none of the women I've talked to—myself included—came to this place overnight. It's been a matter of patience, strategy, analysis, sacrifice. I've been working for myself for thirteen years and it's only within the last few that a lengthy sabbatical has been even remotely possible. All those years before that? A sabbatical was laughable.

And furthermore, maybe you *don't* want a life of endless travel. (The way my anxiety is set up, I require a home base, personally.) Maybe you just want to get through the day without feeling fatigued or to have a career that doesn't make you contemplate running away every three business days.

A break, however long it may be, is about ushering you *out* of survival mode, which requires you to sit still long enough to identify what in your current life is keeping you stuck in the same cycle. We're creatures of comfort. Our nervous system would prefer to keep us in a familiar hell than allow us to venture out into the unknown.

Even if a long-term break may not be in the cards for you right this moment, that doesn't mean we stop our investigation there. We're going to keep daydreaming about the best way to get the rest you deserve, the investment in your well-being that has been eluding you for too long.

MINI SABBATICALS

The Weekender	**A full weekend to breathe and reset. Create an agenda for yourself to hit all the areas you want to cover—do you need some physical replenishment, where you're off your feet and being tended to by warm bathwater? Or do you need a weekend not to be needed by anyone else, where your whims are your own?**
The Primetime	**Send the kids to bed early or simply send them to their room for you to enjoy your quiet brainstorming time. Add in a delicious dinner and a soothing beverage.**
The Holiday	**Holidays usually come with bonus time off. If you have time off with an upcoming holiday, consider making it a low-key affair with as little as possible on your schedule. Don't cook, don't host, don't go all out. Relax.**

Taking a step back to assess requires courage. It may stir up some hard truths about your workload and career path. As you are brainstorming, think of the most you can grant yourself. If a three-month sabbatical is out of reach, is a three-day version possible? One week? A smattering of mental health days spaced throughout the year so each day doesn't feel like a constant grind?

Whatever is accessible to you, claim it. Walk in it. Understand that building a rest ethic is just as, if not more, important than our work ethic. Rest will comfort us when we're tired, replenish us when we're spent, boost us when we're uncertain. Questions to help you craft a sabbatical that works for you:

- What kind of break do I need? Am I feeling run-down mentally, physically, or emotionally?
- Do I need more support in my career and/or my home life? If so, what would make the biggest difference right away?
- Am I feeling seen and supported in my workplace? If not, what would make the biggest difference right away? Do I need a career change?

IMPOSTOR SYNDROME

PSYCHOLOGISTS PAULINE ROSE CLANCE and Suzanne Imes first coined the term "impostor phenomenon" in 1978 after studying 150 high-achieving women—women with doctorates, professional awards, and scholastic honors.[6] It baffled the duo to hear women say things like "I'm not good enough to be on the faculty here" or "Obviously I'm in this position because my abilities have been overestimated." Now dubbed "impostor syndrome," it's most known as the feeling that you're not really as good as your title or accomplishments may suggest.

Most of the women Clance and Imes studied were middle- to upper-class white women under 45. (They found that it was much less likely for men to have impostor syndrome, and when they did, it didn't affect the way they showed up all that much.)

They offered two reasons for why it may occur—both stemming from early childhood experiences of either being compared to the "smart sibling" or having the pressure of holding that title yourself. In the years since their study, more attention has been paid to Black women and impostor syndrome. For us, impostor syndrome can cause self-doubt and hypervigilance, particularly in white-dominated spaces where we are one of a few or an Only. Researchers have found it in every field, from law to business to the arts.

In *Things I Should Have Told My Daughter*, playwright Pearl Cleage shared this journal entry from 1978:[7]

> I am afraid what I am writing is bullshit.
> I am afraid what I am writing is self-indulgent.
> I am afraid what I am writing is of no interest to anyone.
> I am afraid all of it is poorly written.

At the time of this entry, Cleage was 30 years old and a speechwriter for Maynard Jackson, Atlanta's first Black mayor, trying to make the leap to creative writing full-time. Her nerves, on display through much of the process, are classic self-doubt and impostor syndrome. That entry knocked something loose in me as a writer. As Erykah Badu quipped, "I'm an artist and I'm sensitive about my shit." That sensitivity is a hyperawareness that everyone won't rock with what you offer, and what will we do if the majority decide our gift isn't actually a gift at all?

For Cleage, she soon got what she was looking for—she produced her first play three years after that journal entry and went on to enjoy more than forty years of writing plays, novels, and poetry. She taught at Spelman College, ushering in a new class of writers and thought leaders, like author Tayari Jones. Anyone objectively looking at her legacy might wonder why she ever questioned herself.

When I chatted with Baltimore native Claire Dorsey, 95, I was worried a crackly phone line would interfere with what I was sure would be a phenomenal interview. Tech problems solved, she shared how she worked her way up through the Baltimore City School District, eventually becoming principal, a move that shocked her. "I told the superintendent, I've never been an assistant principal. I can't be a principal." She laughs at the memory now. "Wasn't that stupid?"

Fortunately, the superintendent waved off her concerns, telling her that her previous role as district supervisor gave her enough experience to do the job well. But it wasn't just her own concerns that gave her pause. It was external pressure as well. "You have to get over the fact that there's some people who are not happy for you. 'Why did she get this job?' I had nothing to do with getting the job other than working hard."

Dorsey retired after heading three schools as principal.

One theory surrounding Black women and impostor syndrome is that our mere presence in these spaces is counter to the dominant narrative. We're in spaces where all eyes are on us and we feel it.

"They treat Black women, especially in the workplace, like we don't belong there . . . or that we took a more deserving white person's spot," said Jessica Pharm, HR professional and host of *Blackness and the Workplace* podcast. "That's how they tend to treat us, but every Black person I know is well overqualified for the jobs they have."[8]

Music journalist Danyel Smith, whose tenure includes a stint as editor-in-chief at *Vibe* magazine in the 1990s, came into the industry with a homegrown hunger for hip-hop and R&B. She chronicled this hunger in *Shine Bright,* a love letter to Black women vocalists interwoven with her rise as one of the nation's preeminent music writers.

Smith, often working in rooms as one of the few women present, hustled to convey respect to her musical heroes, Black creatives who often weren't seen as vitally important in "mainstream" media. As she gathered bylines and ascending titles on mastheads around the country, she grappled with her untraditional background. Everything she earned was because she "wrote her ass off." Still, doubts about her abilities followed her through her decades-long career.

"I didn't have my BA or MFA in hand until I was in my late thirties," Smith wrote. "Like so many of us, I bounced between achievement and self-stigmatizing sadness. Impostor syndrome and impulsive bravery. I've lost months at a time, even years or more, to rigorously planned self-sabotage and the ensuing self-beatdowns."

In reading Smith's semi-memoir, it's clear her impostor syndrome had nothing to do with talent and more to do with internalizing external chatter and bias. If there's a voice that says you do not belong and you hear it often enough, over time you just might begin to believe it.

Your impostor syndrome may not always be apparent. Most of your day-to-day life, you're cool, calm, confident. You know what you're doing and there's a certain comfort in your skills and abilities.

But then you get a chance for a promotion. Or it's time to negotiate your new job offer. Or you are asked to present at a board meeting. And the sweat starts.

Oh, no, you think to yourself. Am I ready for this?

Clance and Imes made a few suggestions on combating feeling like an impostor—the one that was most notable was being in a community with other women to discuss their feelings. Something about hearing another woman you admire share their feelings of inadequacy snaps you out of your own self-doubt.

I pulled a page from their book when I sat down with *Stop Waiting for Perfect* author L'Oreal Thompson Payton, a writer friend whose similar backstory (Black girls obsessed with magazines with stints at nonprofits before careers as freelancers) made us instantly click.

Payton literally wrote the book on conquering self-doubt. The award-winning journalist's life was already bursting at the seams when the opportunity to write the book came. It was the middle of the coronavirus pandemic, and she was adjusting to new motherhood after several disappointing IVF treatments. *This is terrible timing*, she thought to herself.

She wanted her book to be *right*, she thought, looking at these other authors whose books were seemingly flying off the shelves. "I had a lot of self-doubt and impostor syndrome because who am I to be writing a book, especially a self-help book, if I'm still struggling with the thing I'm trying to help them through?" she told me. "I was trying to emulate other self-help authors that I've seen and their success and lost my voice in the process. The book demanded that I get real and honest and vulnerable about the challenges that I had."

The book-writing process, her biggest career leap yet, helped Payton make peace with impostor syndrome. "I'm constantly having to level up, which means impostor syndrome, for now at least, is going to continue to rear its ugly head. My hope is that people shorten the cycle. So instead of letting impostor syndrome, self-doubt, perfectionism, fear, and all these things sideline you for weeks, maybe instead you're down for the count for two days and you can pick yourself back up and throw your hat in the ring and try again."

Personally, when impostor syndrome creeps up, I call on writer Octavia Butler, whose manifestation of her life's work has inspired me more times than I can count. In her archives, researchers have found her 1988 "So be it, see to it" proclamation in which she declares the following to be true: *This is my life. I write bestselling novels. . . . My books will be read by millions of people. So be it. See to it.*[9]

Her words proved prophetic, with her future novels winning awards and landing her a MacArthur "genius" grant. Her call to herself ("so be it, see to it") is a reminder that we are capable of more than we imagine. Our successes *are* real. They can be *called forth*.

What's impostor syndrome when you know you can co-create with the universe? What's a little self-doubt when you know that you have the power to shift your dreams into reality? What's impostor syndrome when you know that you were born to win?

CHARTING YOUR OWN PATH

"YOUR POSITION HAS been eliminated, effective immediately." Upon hearing those seven words, all the air had been sucked out of the room.

At this point, I was 24 years old, a mom of two kids under 4, and a new homeowner with a new car note in my first semester of graduate school. Money was flowing out of my account faster than I could blink.

Hearing that I no longer had a job (effective immediately, no less) was probably the worst news I could have received after I followed my boss into her office that chilly November afternoon, in the wake of the Great Recession of 2008.

I was stunned. In my mind, going to work every day and putting in a solid effort should have guaranteed that I would be kept on when it came to cutbacks. But it was business, plain and simple.

After I gathered my things and took the slow, agonizing journey to my car, I thought about what this meant. Now that I no longer had to get up every morning and make the hour-long commute to my job, what would I actually do?

I knew I had to hurry up and figure out how to make money. While my husband still had his job, losing my salary meant that paying the mortgage (and several other bills) was going to be a challenge until I could begin to bring in income.

But somehow I knew that this was the chance I had been waiting for: the chance to be self-employed and work full-time for myself.

While I was grateful for all I learned at that organization, I knew there was no room for advancement. As a young Black woman still learning how to move in corporate America, it was daunting to navigate the unspoken rules. *How much could I freestyle this job? How much would I be micromanaged? Do I need to go to these department retreats at my boss's vacation home, designed to give us time to relax together, when I really just wanted to be at home with my kids?* At some point I was going to have to move on, but I hadn't expected to be shoved out the door.

It took some time, but I became convinced that getting laid off was the best thing that could have happened to me. It propelled me into a life I didn't think possible: entrepreneurship.

Black women have been the fastest growing group of entrepreneurs for more than a decade, outpacing every other group.[10] Why are so many of us taking that leap of faith and putting our all into our great business idea? Part of it is the legacy of Black women's entrepreneurial genius. Even as enslaved women, Black women would take advantage of their precious free time, working by candlelight to produce garments and other goods in order to provide income and to hopefully save enough one day to buy their freedom and the freedom of their loved ones. Our legacy of entrepreneurship is deeply embedded and comes with deep cultural pride.

But for all the hard work and sacrifice, the returns look bleak. The majority of Black women lead businesses that earn less than $30,000 in revenue each year.[11] The bulk of us are overworked and underpaid, similar to how we fare in the corporate world, as we work on fixing these numbers.

Of course, as it is with most stats, the numbers only tell part of the story. The fuller story is that Black women tend to self-fund their businesses and lack the same access to start-up capital thanks to bro culture in investment spaces.[12] It takes money to make money.

Entrepreneurs, in order to be well, you need three things—*sufficient funding, a passion for the work,* and *a support system that will rock with you on your business's ups and downs.* You can get pretty far with two of these, but all three is the cheat code.

ADEQUATE FUNDING

Being underpaid was a consistent theme throughout my professional career. I can tell you from personal experience that being underfunded will take you out.

As a consultant, I had no idea what to charge, so I continually priced myself low to keep a steady flow of income, not realizing that by raising my prices, I could do less work for more profit. I did a horrible job negotiating and increasing rates to keep up with the cost of living.

As a product-based business owner, I struggled with too many roles. From sourcing materials, setting pricing, building the website, design, and so on—all of it flowed from my brain to the laptop. I desperately needed help, but my tiny budget was at odds with my ethics of paying people what their time is worth. At one point, I simply created two email accounts on the back end. One was from me, the face of the business. The other was "Chloe," my imaginary assistant, who would respond to customers and promise to send messages up the line to me. I was always terrified that one day I would get them mixed up and send an email from the wrong account, blowing my cover. Why on earth did I do that? I was trying my best to give the appearance of a well-oiled machine, in the hopes of eventually finding a real Chloe. I continued to wear all the hats in my business until I eventually burned out.

Even though Black women overwhelmingly have the entrepreneurial spirit, when we don't have the financial backing to delegate and grow a team right away, we strap on our superwoman cape and get to work anyway.

Nikki Porcher founded Buy from a Black Woman (BFABW) to ensure fewer Black female entrepreneurs shutter their business due to funding issues. She built BFABW as a nonprofit grassroots incubator, providing access to customers, funding, and community support. In the years since its founding, BFABW helped business owners see more than $3 million in revenue.

I first met Porcher and her organization around the time she launched the first Buy from a Black Woman business grant. Porcher put up $250 of her own money, matched with $250 from a board member, to offer one entrepreneur $500 to put toward her business. At the time, it was the first grant I had seen marketed specifically to us. "When you're first starting your business and you're just not sure, and there's nothing like what you have and there's nothing else for Black women, a $500 grant is phenomenal," she told me. "And it is not just a monetary value, it's the validation. There's a stranger out there that sees what I'm doing, they believe in what I'm doing, and they're willing to invest in what I'm doing. So let me keep going."

With two-thirds of us self-funding our business, we must find additional sources to invest in our vision.[13] For Black women, I understand that's more than a notion. Less than 2 percent of venture capital funding goes to companies run by women or people of color. Black venture capitalist Arlan Hamilton, whose firm Backstage Capital has invested more than $30 million into businesses by underrepresented groups, built the company to address the disparity. "We came for the cake, but we're still getting crumbs," she wrote in a Mashable op-ed.[14] "We came for the cake, but once again we're leaving the table hungry."

It's time you get your cake.

If you find yourself financially strapped after self-funding your business, this is your sign to pause and reassess. You deserve to be invested in. You deserve to have an ample budget to be able to build your business the way you desire. Apply to any and all grants. Get connected at your local Small Business Administration office. Establish or fix your business credit so you can apply for loans to support your goals.

The main question is: *How much of my headache and stress is be-*

cause I am trying to bootstrap this enterprise? For most of us, a blank check would solve a world of stress. Ensuring we can be well means we have to look at the reality of our bank account. Either you find the funding to operate the business at the level you desire or you right-size your project to fit the budget you have. But making *yourself* the stopgap that solves your financial problems, is putting yourself in the fast lane to burnout. You deserve a business that supports *you*.

WHERE'S THE JOY?

My network is full of people who are committed to doing business differently. Best example? India Pierce, the "Joy Ambassador." After years of working in the DEI space, she's made a conscious choice to center joy in her work.

Pierce, 35, launched a luxury picnic business, where she'd create these lavish physical vignettes for customers. A little while later, she began to experiment with her own agency as the CEO. "Once I was setting up a picnic at the beach, and we were in the sand. I was like, *This is not a part of my joyful business plan.* And immediately stopped doing beach picnics and just recognized the freedom that had come with me creating boundaries and being okay with it. Not feeling like I was missing out on anything. Running that business taught me a lot in terms of what it looks like to just unapologetically do what I want to do, and to not let money dictate the moves that I make."

At this point in our conversation I had to confess that what she was suggesting—walking away from potential income—took me *years* to fully practice.

"When I really sat down to think about *what is my joyful vision for my life*, spaciousness is what kept coming up for me," Pierce told me. "And I can't have spaciousness if I'm running three businesses.

I recognized I was in that tilling phase of my life where I was trying to pick up and turn over the soil and get some air in there and figure out what needed to go, to pull out the weeds and to get ready to plant new seeds."

Other entrepreneurs I interviewed had the same come-to-Jesus moment with themselves, where it became apparent that they needed a new mode of business.

"Nothing will burn you out more than building a business that you don't even like," Alicia Robertson said. "You may make some money, but it's gonna be stressful. You're not gonna enjoy it. That's what's gonna lead you to burnout more than working eighty hours a day."

Robertson speaks from personal experience. After coaching entrepreneurs for close to a decade, she began to feel a gentle tug that something about her business model was off. "I went to therapy. I was able to get on a medication that really helped with a lot of the anxiety and day-to-day depression. I started working out more. And while those things were helping a lot, it was still the business part that wasn't sustainable."

She switched from individual to group coaching, thinking it was enough change to bring the relief she was seeking. It wasn't. "I would get onto these coaching calls and I would feel frustrated. I would feel annoyed. My clients were great; they were fine. I just did not want to do it."

She eventually shut down her coaching business entirely, getting a full-time job as a community manager. Pivoting to full-time employment, with someone else worrying about the bottom line for a year, gave Robertson the break she needed to figure out how entrepreneurship would work best for her. Now she's back with a community-based offering, where there's space for community members to assist each other, giving her room to be the lead but not the sole knowledgeable voice in the room.

Robertson has a few questions for the weary entrepreneur (Is that you, sis?): "Is the business you're building, is that something you actually want to do? Are these people actually people you want to help? Are these services leaving you fulfilled or are they leaving you drained? When different trends pop up online, people want to try all of these new things or build all these new businesses based on someone else's idea of success—they forget what they actually want to do."

Like Pierce and Robertson, locating the source of your passion keeps you tethered to the larger picture.

BUSINESS BESTIES

Andrea Butler, 43, is the former editor-in-chief of *Sesi* magazine, which for many years was the only print magazine for Black teen girls in the United States. We met while attending the same predominately white journalism program, where I was an undergrad and she was in grad school. Our connection remained after she graduated and moved three states away. At some point (neither of us can remember how we started), we began having what we called our "vision chats."

Between my life as a mom of two and hers as an EIC, we had to pull out the calendars to figure out what would work best. We settled on the third Monday of the month for an hour-long call updating each other on everything that's going on in our lives. I vent, then she vents, then we eventually circle back around to look at the bright side of things and give each other a word of encouragement before we head back to our lives for another month.

We have held these calls consistently since 2014. She is the most consistent part of my friendship circle because I know, barring a natural disaster or major emergency, every third Monday of the month we're going to be chatting, releasing our pent-up anger or laughing until we cry.

She helps problems become "figureoutable." Without these consistent calls, I would be spinning my wheels. She's a safe space for my business failures and frustrations. She's seen me shut down my subscription box business due to overwhelm and stalemates with shipping partners; I consoled her when she had to shutter her magazine. It's easy to find people who will celebrate your wins with you. It's quite another to find people who are ready to walk through the mud with you.

That support is crucial for Black women business owners, who are historically trying to do more with less.

"People are realizing, *I cannot work in a silo anymore*. I cannot do this on my own," Porcher told me. "They realize, I've been doing so much on my own, but in order to get what's next I need community. And that's community that's building with you, community that's holding you accountable. Community with your future peers that you want to grow into and look like."

As Issa Rae once said, "Network across. Who's next to you? Who's struggling? Who's in the trenches with you? Who's just as hungry as you are? And those are the people that you need to build with."[15]

Building as a solopreneur is a lonely endeavor. Building our network allows us the space to hear new ideas, release pent-up frustration, or otherwise have a listening ear when we need some feedback.

Sometimes we like to keep quiet about our aspirations out of fear: *What if I tell people about this goal and I fail? I'll look foolish.*

Truthfully, every idea won't work out. Oprah doesn't have a thirty-year winning streak. She's had some very public failures. Everybody has. What counts is that you got up there and tried to do something. It's easier to navigate those leaps when you've got people on board who want to see you soar.

Success awaits.

TEND TO YOUR PROFESSIONAL WELLNESS

EVERY OTHER CHAPTER of this book gives you the tools to be your best so you can bring your best self to your career. Here's a few items that belong front of mind when we're considering how to move through your professional career—however long or short it is—with grace:

SET REASONABLE PROJECT DEADLINES

I share this in the spiritual wellness chapter: *You are one human person.* Take the time to think about what you can reasonably handle, considering any possible obstacles or setbacks. When each step is reasonable, you feel happy with your progress and you can make the bigger leaps (from a rough draft to a finished book, for example) much easier.

BE BRAVE WHEN YOU GOTTA BE BRAVE

Sometimes you need to do something before you *know* you can do something. And that's scary, yes. We all get scared when we're called out of our comfort zones and asked to soar. But there's a reason you're called to do this. There's growth and joy and beauty on the other side of your bravery. Leap.

MARK YOUR PROGRESS

Having mini milestones is important because you see that all those late nights actually mean something and you're not grinding just because. This goes back to #1 (setting reasonable deadlines). You want to stay motivated and enthused about your progress. Give yourself a reason to keep going!

MAKE "GROWTH" YOUR MANTRA

When there are setbacks in my business, I do not crumble. I do not fold. Instead, I lean into those failures and find the lesson. Should I have been more proactive? Is there a system I should put in place next time I'm confronted with a similar situation? Should I have brought in a partner? Learning those lessons takes the sting out of setbacks and keeps you motivated to try again another day.

TILLING THE SOIL: PROFESSIONAL WELLNESS JOURNALING QUESTIONS

- What do I need to release in my relationship with work?
- How can I center my well-being in my weekly work schedule?
- What is missing in my career that would bring me copious amounts of joy?
- Am I feeling un(der)supported?
- Where do I see my career headed in the next five years? Are there steps I need to take now to get me there?

Fill Me Up

SPIRITUAL WELLNESS

I tell people all the time—we're a church for grown people. I don't micromanage people's relationship with Christ. I give you tools to figure out what it needs to look like for you and God. I've even moved away from the language of "church" and I've been actually trying to move towards the term "sacred community." We recognize that God is in the midst of us, but God is also in the midst of each of us. And I am our leader, but I'm not especially special. Does that make sense? I'm trying to figure it out for me too. And all I can do is give you the tools to do that.

—Pastor Courtney Clayton Jenkins, 42

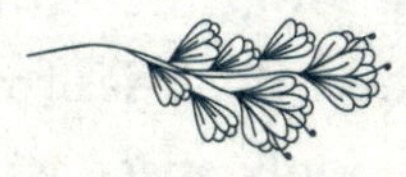

EXPLORING THE ROOTS

ONE SLEEPY SUNDAY in church, I catch a glimpse of what I imagine to be an example of holy sisterhood in action: A woman two rows ahead of me feels the beginnings of a hot flash. I watch as she leans forward and grabs the visitor information index card from the pew pocket in front of her and tries to fan herself with the small rectangle, to no avail.

No more than ten seconds later, she feels a tap on the shoulder. A fellow attendee offers up a hand fan, some sweet relief for her "personal summer." She grasps her sister's hand in gratitude for a moment and puts her wrist to work to cool off.

Crisis averted.

The tender moment between two Black women gathered to hear their weekly dose of praise and worship stuck with me for months. Is there anything more beautiful or spiritual than being in need and having someone come to your aid, giving you just what you need, an unspoken prayer being answered?

Indeed, the Black Church—traditionally Christian and male-led—has historically been the most consistent source of strength and renewal for Black women, who pack its pews every week to receive a word in their Sunday best.

Above all, Black women *believe.* As the most religious group in America (97 percent of us believe in some form of a higher power[1]), our faith is as loud as it is long-standing. Our numbers aren't surprising as you consider our history and the necessity of faith in our most desperate hours. From the earliest days in America, the enslaved had one space where their desires, words, prayers could be honored—the church. The only space where the rules were theirs to shape and define, the only place their agency was honored. Praising their way through horror in the hopes that tomorrow would bring liberation, or at the very least, the strength to endure. That persistent, dogged faith is a generational heirloom.

If Black women do anything, we go to church. As I sat with Gardeners over the years, faith was a constant through our conversations, steeped in most of their memories.

"Baby, I'm 69 years old," Colette Hill of Cleveland said, laughing. "If we didn't go to church on Sunday, something was extremely wrong with this picture. Grew up in the church from a baby. Like how you wash your face and brush your teeth every day? Going to church was like that. Unless you were sick or dying, you were in church every Sunday."

However, in all areas of American life, formal religion is at a crossroads.[2] Attendance is down, tithes are falling. The average American is less active in church than their predecessors, Black folks included. With each passing year, the number of religiously unaffiliated grows, with those in religious communities stressing about where the next generation of churchgoers will come from.

For all the hand-wringing, I consider this moment a glorious opportunity to get reacquainted with our spiritual selves. We've never lost touch with our inner spiritual guide because it's always there, like our breath. But just like our breath, if we don't pay attention to it, we find ourselves going shallow instead of deep. We miss out on that restoration.

I'm well aware that we all come to this conversation with a varied spiritual background, but one thing that binds us is our spiritual self, that piece of us that transcends this physical body.

When we talk about spiritual wellness, we're not strictly talking about practicing *religion*, the structured approach to the connection to the divine, the doctrines and the dogma. In this chapter, we're focusing on *spirituality*, which is broader than religion and focused more on the individual's relationship with all things soulful.

You ever hear someone say "I'm spiritual, not religious"? Usually it's code for "I don't go to church but Jesus/Yahweh/Jehovah is all right with me." But truthfully, even within whatever religion you practice (or if that's no religion at all), your spiritual walk can exist outside of Sunday morning sermons and Bible study.

Knowing the stats about Black women and religion, you undoubtedly have some familial influence in who and what you worship. Whether your folks dragged you to church every Sunday or you never saw the inside of a church your entire childhood, the good news is you are able to design a spiritual walk that makes sense to you. Of all the facets of wellness we discuss in this book, this is the most personal work you can encounter, because it literally leads us to consider what it means to be human. At our core, who are we? What do we believe? How do we want to move through this one precious life?

It's a tall order. To guide us, our relationship with our spiritual selves can be broken down into four categories:

Within self—What do you know to be true about yourself? How do you move in relationship to what you need? What do you tell yourself about yourself?

Within our relationship with others—How do we love those closest to us and those who have come before us?

Within nature—What do we believe about our relationship to nature that's all around us? How do we engage and care for the planet where we reside?

With the divine—Is there a higher power that we rely on to help us through life's turbulence? How do we connect with its omnipresence?

Once we grapple with and answer these questions, then we're ready for a robust spiritual walk that guides us when we get weary and comforts us when we need its embrace.

WHO TAUGHT YOU ABOUT SPIRITUALITY?

WHEN I THINK of church, I think of candy.

As a child, sitting through marathon church services tested my attention span. My father would slip me and my sisters peppermints at regular intervals to provide just enough of a sugar rush to keep us from going feral. In other cases I'd scribble on an envelope from the back pew pocket to occupy my mind during a service that just wasn't hitting home yet. Our postchurch ritual of "getting something good to eat" kept me focused on the sermon just enough to get through to the fried chicken, rice, and gravy that awaited me at Old Country Buffet. (Don't judge us!)

Those long services (which, looking back, probably weren't as long as I remember) were my entry to the African Methodist Episcopal tradition.

For more than forty years, if anyone asked my parents where they went to church, they would answer: "I go to Lee."

Lee Memorial AME sits on East 105th Street in Cleveland, one of eight churches in a one-mile stretch. The brick building nestled itself on the corner of a residential street, with its stained glass windows and steep brick stairs to lead you inside. When I visit it now, I'm always surprised by how small it is. It felt cavernous as a child, with its hard oak pews and massive altar that most modern churches have swapped for an open-air, accessible space.

You can trace my family history through that church—my parents were married there in 1984, I married my husband in its "new building" in 2007, and my children were both christened at its altar in the following two years. I've only attended a handful of services since going away to college, but every time I come back, it is utterly familiar. It feels like home.

For forty-one of its one hundred years in existence, Rev. Wesley I. Reid was head pastor of the midsize congregation. His sermons were animated, lively, full of "I won't be before you longs" that almost certainly meant he's going to be before us long. For most of my attendance, Lee Memorial was predominantly female, and yet I don't recall many Black women in the pulpit, outside of the occasional Women's Day speaker. Through my early church experiences, I learned that *when it comes to spiritual matters, women are present yet sidelined.*

As much as I was able to receive from Reverend Reid every week, I wonder how it would have shaped me to see a Black woman delivering her investigation into God's word. Would I have been more engaged seeing a Black woman share her thoughts on what it meant to live a good and righteous life? Would I have needed the candy?

What are women missing when the primary voice between us and God is male? While I have no doubt that male pastors can and should be preaching to the entire congregation, I can only report that I have been the most fed being in conversation with other Black women. In so many areas of our life, our preference often skews female—with our gynecologists, our hairstylists, our nail techs. There is an inherent understanding. It makes sense that a feminine approach to spirituality might feed us more.

Without realizing it, I had been seeking a womanist bent to my faith walk. Womanist theology—the consideration of gender, race, racism, sexism, and power within theological frameworks[3]—sprung from Alice Walker's *womanist* definition from 1983:[4]

> A woman who loves other women, sexually and/or nonsexually. Appreciates and prefers women's culture, women's emotional flexibility . . . and women's strength. . . . Committed to survival and wholeness of entire people, male and female. Not a separatist, except periodically, for health. . . . Loves music. Loves dance. Loves the moon. Loves the Spirit . . . Loves struggle. Loves the folk. Loves herself. Regardless. Womanist is to feminist as purple is to lavender.

I wanted to know exactly what God sees for me as a Black woman. How do I construct a faith journey that fills me up and recognizes the path I walk?

Author Yolanda Pierce wrote the book on Black women and faith. *In My Grandmother's House: Black Women, Faith, and the Stories We Inherit* could be described as a literary monument to Pierce's grandmother, a woman of such tremendous faith that "in a different generation she probably would've been a minister."[5]

Pierce takes womanist theology one step further and introduces "grandmother theology," honoring the women who've come before us and shaped our faith.

"When I think about the image of the divine, it should invoke love, safety, comfort, connection, and joy," Pierce said in an interview. "In the earthly realm, I experienced that in my grandmother's house. My grandmother's house is where I found safety, an expression of God, and the holy."

Pierce believes Black women have, for too long, been relegated to being the church's backbone, when our gifts and talents have been apparent and ready for the pulpit. Even now, as I write this, Black women account for one-half of Black masters' students in seminary, but less than 10 percent of church leadership.[6]

My paternal aunt, the Reverend Felicia Hopkins, is one of the few to reach the top. Having been ordained in the United Methodist Church since 1996, her tenure has been filled with highs and lows.

She's preached in front of congregations of all demographics: majority white, majority Black, mixed. One thing remains constant: "I'm here to give you the Word," she told me. "Along the way I have learned and been coached how to effectively deliver that word without losing my authenticity."

My talk with her reminds me that we must always bring our full self to our faith spaces. As a Black woman, what do you see? How does your faith anchor your identity? Or maybe I should ask: How does your identity anchor your faith?

An elder millennial Christian, I now find myself straddling the traditions of old and the innovation of new. You can catch me in church quite a few Sundays out of the year, but I stay busy interrogating my faith outside of weekly church services. I pray. I do yoga. I listen to gospel. I write my annual goals on a prayer candle and light it whenever I am working on my goal. I gather with my friends as we try to figure out the best way to move through these increasingly complex lives with some sense of grace. Above all, I try to be exceptionally good to people and thoroughly kind and gentle with myself. All these things together give me peace and a connection to God.

WHO TAUGHT YOU ABOUT SPIRITUALITY?

- What were you taught about organized religion? Is it vital to your spiritual wellness to be a formal member of a congregation?
- If you regularly attended religious services as a child, what do you remember about it? What was your favorite part? What, if anything, was missing?
- Have there been any deviations in your family's religious history? Has anyone converted or made any sharp turns in their spiritual journey?
- Can you identify any aspects of your spiritual rituals that you picked up from your parental figures? Think gospel music, candles, prayers, and so on.
- What limitations exist for you as a spiritual person? Do you refrain from cursing, self-pleasure, alcohol, and such as a matter of religious principle?
- Have you ever been curious about a religion other than the one you were raised in?
- What sources (books, people, other media) guide your spiritual walk?

RELATIONSHIP WITH SELF
Granting Self-Compassion

WHEN WOMEN REQUEST to join The Self Care Suite, I ask them their biggest obstacle when it comes to self-care. The women are surprisingly candid and vulnerable, offering, "I don't know how to make time for myself" or "I'm terrible at setting boundaries," along with a quick story of how they know this to be true.

But overwhelmingly, the most common admission is the prevailing guilt that accompanies them through every attempt to make life easier for themselves.

Where did this guilt come from?

I firmly believe guilt is a scam. It's manufactured by the majority culture. It's carefully honed, generation after generation, in order to produce generations of women whose entire identity is wrapped up in being a support for others. When Zora Neale Hurston wrote that Black women are the mules of the world, she told no lie.[7]

That guilt is a reminder that you have forgotten how holy you are. You've forgotten how much you deserve. There's more for you. Time to claim it.

Your relationship with yourself is a spiritual endeavor. The way you talk about yourself, what you tolerate, what you believe about yourself—all of that is an indication of how you feel about the vessel you were blessed with.

Feeling guilty is one of the first things we tackle in our self-care workshops, because if you can't grab hold of the truth of what you deserve, we can't go any further. Your higher power designed you to shine, to unequivocally declare, "This is mine. And I'm taking it."

(Don't believe in a higher power? Regardless of your beliefs, you are the product of generations that came before you and the community that stands beside you. They all want to see you win.)

When I don't tend to myself like I should, when I don't offer myself enough grace, I'm lacking in self-compassion. When we believe that we are somehow performing below or outside of expectations (whether our own or societal), we feel guilt for not being able to match it. We turn that shame inward, and our internal dialogue starts to sound a little like this:

Am I giving enough time to my kids? Are they eating too much junk food? Are they learning enough? Am I doing enough to tend to their emotional, mental, and physical needs? Hell, am I giving enough attention to myself? I'm so tired.

We've got to find a calm space in the center of all this, and self-compassion is the thing that'll get us there.

Dr. Kristin Neff, who literally wrote the book on self-compassion, defines it in three parts: *self-kindness, common humanity, and mindfulness.*[8]

Self-kindness. When things don't go quite our way, we're still able to be warm and gracious toward ourselves.

Common humanity. Humans mess up sometimes. We all feel a bit inadequate in certain situations.

Mindfulness. Being an observer of our emotions (*Ah, that's sadness. Hm, that's anger.*) allows us to not overly identify with the emotions from our pain or disappointment.

It bears repeating—wrestling with what it means to be human is to embrace the mess that lives within us all. Our higher power did not create humans with perfect operating systems and predictable patterns. That same power gave us all a limit, a capacity for how much we can successfully manage on any given day. A large portion of strengthening your spiritual walk is learning how to treat yourself like the human—and spiritual being—you are.

Next time you find yourself at war with yourself, hear this: Treat yourself with the knowledge that you are a spiritual being having a human experience. You are one of one.

RELATIONSHIP WITH SELF
Cultivating Hope

CULTIVATING A STRONG "hope ethic" is the work of a lifetime. Our proximity to bad news is the closest and most consistent it's ever been—with one tap of the screen we can be informed of everything that's going on in any corner of the world, with headlines ranging from mild to atrocious. There's cell phone footage putting us right at the scene, denying us the privilege of looking away even if we tried. That type of forced awareness can take a toll on our mental health and ability to hope. *Is every day going to be like this?* we start to wonder.

Simply willing ourselves to "think positive" might work in the short term but it's not a sustainable strategy.

So what might we try? Radical acceptance.

Of course, we wake up and pray that everything goes well—all green lights on the way to work, donuts in the break room, an unexpected flower delivery when we get home, and our partner telling us, "Don't worry, I'll cook tonight." And sometimes we will have days like this, where all seems right in the world. But that "hope ethic" really comes into play when the day is not so great, when it's harder to be optimistic.

Radical acceptance is understanding that humanity is *messy*. Life will make us cry, make us think, make us cuss. It's climbing the mountain. It's withstanding the waves. It's arduous *and* fulfilling. Because life isn't meant to be impossible, but it is meant to make us grow. It's not always hard, but it ain't always easy. Most days fall in the balance between the two. Having hope means you know things can get better.

With such big issues facing us (white supremacy, climate change, threats to democracy, to name a few), it may not feel like "hope" is enough. But consider what remains if you take hope away. How do you wake up and face each day if there's no small part of you that believes things can possibly change?

Professor Tiya Miles reminds us that Blackness *is* hopefulness: "The capacity to recognize those moments of emergency, catastrophe and impending loss as moments of change and then to anticipate what might come next are part of the psychological and emotional tool kit that saved Black America."[9]

Our biggest cultural inheritance is hope. We originated "making a way outta no way." We invented all forms of music—spirituals, the blues, rap—that allowed us to express angst while we fight for better.

Nothing fortified my hope ethic like spending three years immersed in interviews with one hundred Black women. Not surprisingly, I got to hear about the realities of race and civil rights from women in their fifties and up. Common stories of not being expected to go to college, or, once they got there, finding a hostile environment. Something as simple as not being able to sit where you want to at the movie theater (if you were even allowed to go in) or being relegated to mopping the floors in homes you would never afford to live in.

They told me such incredible stories of resilience, of displaying strength they shouldn't have had to wield. But there was also so much *joy* in their stories. Their lives were filled with community, laughter, and faith. Despite the challenges, they still carved out a meaningful life. Sitting with my elders—my friends' grandmothers, church ladies, cousins, neighbors— widened my perspective. Since starting these interviews, I'm a bit calmer while handling the ebbs and flows of life. *They did it. I can do it too, I hope.*

You don't have to interview one hundred people, but the act of sitting with your elders is a life-changing one. It reminds you that you are not the first person to encounter a setback, a denial, or world-shifting headlines. You can persevere, in some cases easier than those who came before you, because they can tell you what worked, what didn't, what they wished they had done differently. You can move knowing you are standing on the shoulders of giants. Your hope ethic isn't just for you, but for everyone who came before you as well.

If all else fails, wellness advocate and podcast host Francheska Medina shared a two-word practice for cultivating hope: *Zoom out.* I tend to move toward catastrophic thinking (re: *everything* is a potential crisis) and I've realized it just doesn't serve me to spend my energy this way. So in those moments where I feel so overwhelmed and afraid and worn out, I try my best to zoom out:

- What am I missing in my perspective?
- What additional information should I consider?

- Is this a problem for someone other than me to solve?
- Who can I call in to help me problem solve?

Sometimes hope lies in the details you can't see when you're eye to eye with the problem at hand. Sometimes zooming out is your best line of defense in maintaining your hope.

RELATIONSHIP WITH SELF
Traveling Through Time

I SPEND SEVERAL hours a week loving on and talking to my 20-year-old Self. It is this age that my lifelong anxiety began to manifest more externally, going from a quiet hum to a piercing scream. A college junior, she just found out she's pregnant and now she's terrified of the future, worried that she won't be able to simultaneously nurture both a baby and a writing career. Only pregnant for a few weeks and she had to make big decisions already: She just turned down her dream internship with *Essence* magazine, not having enough money to spend the summer in New York without coming home broke. She's scared this is where her story ends. Having seen the next twenty chapters, I can wrap my arms around her and rock her with confidence.

"Baby you are going to be a phenomenal mother and writer," I tell her, wiping tears off her cheeks. "Your baby girl is in college now. She's happy and thriving. And hey, don't freak out but you had another baby too. Yeah, about two years from now. A boy! He's a phenomenal kid. And guess what? You do indeed write a book. Several!"

I picture her lifting her head to look at me. "Really?"

"Really," I assure her. "Just do what you know how to do. It all falls into place."

These conversations (think of it as time traveling) bring that "Write a letter to your younger self" exercise to life. I stumbled upon this practice when doing some journaling to my past self. With perspective and time, I was able to write her a letter to let her know that she did the best she could with the information she had, and I was proud of her for making tough decisions. In some way, I know she received it at the right moment.

This practice allows you to see you as your higher power or as loved ones see you. As a person simply trying to get through life. Your only job at that moment is to offer love. No judgment. No scolding. But love. Love without conditions, without a wish to go back and change things. (As every time traveling movie has shown us, we can't meddle in the past without repercussions.)

I spend a lot of time with all my past selves.

I tell my 16-year-old Self: "There's much better love waiting for you in the future."

I tell my 25-year-old Self: "You're so brave to strike out and be an entrepreneur, but please remember to take care of yourself first. You're priceless and can't be replaced."

I tell my 35-year-old Self: "Get back to work on that book proposal. The timing is better than you think."

Each version of yourself—the shy teen, the confused 20-something, the more mature 30-year-old—remains with you long after the birthday candles are blown out. They could use that love and support and guidance from you. I'm glad they're still living and existing somewhere within my universe.

Usually when people attempt to time travel with their past selves, they instinctively pick the age they needed the most support or they felt the loneliest. The beauty is when you go back to that time period, you're able to give yourself the love and support you weren't able to receive or give yourself in real time. Only *this* time, there is someone who knows exactly how you're feeling, who knows exactly what you need to hear, and they know exactly how things are going to turn out. And you're able to comfort you in that moment. How divine.

You can do it in either direction. Pick an age in the future. As I write this, I'm 38. I'm imagining 55-year-old Me. I'm looking to her for guidance and reassurance, as I'm nervous about what life will look like for my kids as they embark on their adult journeys.

Imagine if she told me: "We just had Thanksgiving. Both the kids came. They brought the dessert. They're doing so well. They're happy. You did good." That calms me and soothes me. I believe her. I needed confirmation from someone who can tell me, and *I believe her.* Being able to visualize myself in the future—successful, happy, free—allows me to move through today with confidence.

We form in layers. Each version of yourself is a piece of your spirit looking for love, belonging, and support. This practice is about loving all the selves that live within you and making sure they're tended to just as much as your present self, who is just an amalgamation of those former versions. Loving *them* is your number one job.

How can YOU LOVE ON YOU?

- **Write a letter to your future self.** I write an email to myself every January 1 and schedule it to be sent December 31. In it, I detail how proud I am of myself for pressing through another year. Each year when it arrives in my inbox (every single year I forget—ha!) I tear up with love from my past self. She loves me so much.

RELATIONSHIP WITH SELF
Adopting a Slower Pace

TAKING YOUR TIME is a spiritual practice.

During our interview, pastor Courtney Clayton Jenkins recommended a book to me: John Mark Comer's *The Ruthless Elimination of Hurry.* I jotted down the title and downloaded it almost immediately after we hung up.

Comer, a pastor who stepped down at his megachurch to hear his creator more clearly, wrote an entire manifesto on slowing *alllll* the way down. Our overstuffed lives are making us spiritually empty, he argued. "Hurry is violence on the soul."[10]

He took a sabbatical and spent a year coming back to himself, eventually realizing that busyness "cuts off your connection to God, to other people, and even to your own soul."

In a world where we have so much vying for our attention, slowing down is a sign that we trust in life's unfolding. We are calm. We are grounded. We know our path is divinely ordered. Your slower pace says to the universe, "I am exactly where I need to be."

One snowy morning, I was rushing to get my son off to preschool and got my first lesson in taking my time.

Perhaps foolishly, I sat my son down at the bottom of the stairs by the front door and placed his shoes by his feet. "Put those on," I instructed. "I'll be right back. I'm going to warm up the car."

Less than five minutes later I came back inside to find my son sitting on the floor, still fumbling with his shoes. Instead of opening the Velcro first, he was simply trying to shove his feet in, which was taking much longer than I anticipated.

I must have sighed or signaled my impatience in some way. "Mommy, you're always rushing me," he said in annoyance. He pointed a finger at me. "You know where you belong? *Mount Rushmore!*"

If my kids inherited anything from me, it's my love of a good joke, so his Mount Rushmore punch line made me chuckle, despite my annoyance. (And really, I was impressed. Who told him about Mount Rushmore and how did he remember it well enough to get me?) From that moment on, my son's words echoed in my head whenever I was operating at a frenzied pace. I pictured myself on Mount Rushmore, alongside three other moms who just wanted their kids to put their shoes on faster.

But why was I rushing in the first place? What difference did it really make if he took five minutes or six minutes on his shoes? Was my life that structured that an extra minute would have killed me?

Obviously not. But with the perspective of time, I can see that I was rushing because it was simply my default. You know the same dopamine hit you get when you beat the time GPS tells you it will take to get somewhere? I was chasing that same high in my everyday life, trying to squeeze a minute here, a minute there off my tasks so

I could then . . . do the next thing. I too often found myself jetting from task to task, moving at an unsustainable pace. Why?

Maybe because I was trying to fit forty-eight hours into twenty-four. Because I have felt "behind" for over a decade and I have convinced myself that *today* is the day I can catch up. Maybe because I had too much on my plate and instead of looking to see where I could ease up, I was trying to expand my appetite. I needed to slow down. A body perpetually "rushing" is a body searching for calm.

But I am a single mother, I can hear you saying. *I'm a caregiver to my parents. I'm busy at work. I'm a student who is doing her best to graduate on time. My life doesn't allow for a leisurely pace!*

Whatever framing you have of your life is yours. I won't sit here and argue you down that you have all the time in the world to move at a pace that pleases your soul.

I know you're doing your best.

I also know that you're tired. Not that "take a nap and feel refreshed" kind of fatigue. But the kind of fatigue that settles into your bones, makes you groan as you open your eyes in the morning because you know you're going into a new day at a deficit already.

Consider this: What's likely to happen if, next time you catch yourself rushing, you pause, center yourself with a deep breath, then begin again, at a slower, more manageable pace?

More than likely you'll find a stronger feeling that you run the pace of your day, and the pace of the day doesn't run you.

Let that settle.

The first major antidote to rushing is recognizing that your to-do list will never be complete. Your to-do list is not really even a list. It's a cycle. There will always be something on it. Laundry, cooking, cleaning, emailing, driving somewhere . . . it's simply a part of life. That feeling of being "done" is an impossible goal. There's only space in between tasks. That's it.

Once you internalize that, *boom*. The whole world opens. You cease to be one of those people who can't relax until the kitchen is clean because you recognize that the kitchen will be dirty again tomorrow. You calm down about getting all the laundry clean at the same time because you recognize that you wear clothes every day and having clean clothes just means you're at a different place in the cycle. You don't fret about being in the faster line at the grocery store because you're at the grocery store all the time and if you average it out, you pick the faster line 70 percent of the time.

The second antidote is recognizing that you are only one human person. I love knowing there is a "bottom" to my capacity. I love knowing just how much I can accomplish at any given time. It makes me focus on efficiency. I say "yes" to the things that really matter and say "no" to the things that truly don't require my presence or input. I don't kid myself into thinking I can do it all, every day, by myself and still function well. Folks forget that we Black women are mere mortals. It's nothing to ask an overburdened Black woman to give a little more. Committing to a slower pace means I lean all the way in to my humanity.

The Slow DOWN

Meals—How many times have you looked down at your plate and realized, *Dang, did I even taste the food?* Spend time with the meal you spent time preparing.

Conversations—Slow down when talking to the people you love and care about. Do your best to give them undivided attention.
Your literal pace—Whether you're walking through the grocery store or the office, catch yourself if you're moving fast. Ground yourself and breathe. Take your time.
Decision-making—Rushing into giving an answer is the best way to keep your people-pleasing tendencies alive! Pause for yourself and think it through.

A powerful question to ask as you're going about your day: *Why am I rushing?* Catch yourself when you're moving faster than you need to, hustling for reasons you can't identify.

We are singular beings with a finite amount of energy each day. Too many of us are borrowing from tomorrow's energy to get through today, which means we're running a perpetual deficit. I want better for you, dear reader. Practice a slower pace and allow your natural rhythm to become steady and deliberate.

RELATIONSHIPS WITH OTHERS
On the Shoulders of Giants

TO GIVE MYSELF some focus and clarity in the countdown to Election Day 2016, I turned off MSNBC and CNN and took to immersing myself in genealogy research. I spent hours on ancestry websites, reading old yearbook captions, and saving photos of my family members from the 1930s, becoming a pro at deciphering old census records.

In the midst of uncertainty, I needed a reminder of who I am, of the generations of people who built families that would one day become my bloodline.

I needed to pull on their knowledge, their wisdom, their strength, their courage. My blood is their blood and I needed to hear them whisper to me, "Baby girl, you doing all right."

I started with my maternal grandma, Marietta Williams, who has always been my favorite person. In every photo of the two of us, from my toddler years to teens, I am glued to her side, smiling wide and happy to be existing in her orbit. She passed on while I was in high school. I miss her terribly. But her strength and her mother's strength and *her* mother's strength are still embedded in me. They keep me going. I am the sum of their prayers, and the lessons they've imparted will never ever leave me.

One example: I spent time on Google Maps recently looking at her old house on Street View and I immediately teared up.

My grandma asked me, when I was 6 or 7, what color she should paint her house. She laid two paint samples in front of me. I told her, with confidence, I liked yellow with green trim.

It is still, to this day, yellow with green trim.

Every time I see the house, I think of the gift she gave me—the proof that my opinion mattered, even as a child.

After my grandmother passed in 2001, she visited me in a dream shortly after her funeral with a message that she was doing well and enjoying her new "home." We hugged, and when I woke, I was filled with the kind of peace that usually only arrives years into the grieving process. I knew I had been in communication with her spirit. I was so grateful that our connection didn't end when she transitioned.

I didn't realize it then, but I started practicing my own form of ancestral veneration soon after. Ancestral veneration (not to be confused with ancestral worship) is the practice of honoring your ancestors, allowing them to retain all the dignity and influence they held while on earth.

What does ancestral veneration look like for me? It looks like finding photos of my ancestors from family members and placing them around the house. It looks like naming my daughter after my sisters. It looks like nurturing the plants I receive from different family funerals. It tastes like baking my late mother-in-law's pound cake recipe on holidays. It feels like wearing my grandmother's necklaces as bracelets to my speaking engagements. It looks like honoring the family that I still have in this realm by asking them to tell their stories.

This spiritual practice is not just about me—it's a communal experience. It's finding where I fit in this complex quilt of DNA. Most spiritualists will define spirituality as an individual relationship between you and a higher power. My spirituality is about the creation of all things divine.

That spiritual connection tethers Aneesah McGregor, 43, when she needs to feel grounded. "Growing up Catholic, everything was so defined on heaven and hell. You do bad things? That's where you're going. It's very fear-based. This really cannot be it. So I started to figure out things that I actually could point to, to ground me. And that's how I started with ancestral veneration. I can actually say that my ancestors were strong and resilient and have strength, because I'm here, I'm a testament to that. My ancestors . . . that's who's carrying me, who's walking with me, who's pushing me forward. Because clearly without that I wouldn't be here."

McGregor doesn't have a traditional altar or space, but she calls on her ancestors for strength.

"The more I think you learn about yourself and your history, all the things that happen, not just in this country, but across the world to people who look like us, you really have to recognize the importance of how strong and resilient we are as people. And I feel like there's magic in that."

Some Christian critics frown on ancestral veneration, pointing to Exodus 20 ("Thou shall have no other gods before me") as proof that God, in His almighty wisdom, requires us to restrict our worship to Him alone. But other theologians push back, arguing that veneration is separate from worship, and that instances of God asking us to honor our ancestors can be found throughout the Bible. My conscience has always been clear, as ancestral veneration isn't placing our foremothers on a pedestal, making them deities. The distinction is in the name—*veneration* is to lend great deference, to honor. It is no more "worship" to honor your ancestors than it is to honor your children. That same chapter in Exodus asks us to exalt our mother and father. Clearly the Christian God believes in familial reverence.

In a viral blog post, Danyelle Thomas, 35, explained how ancestral veneration serves her spiritual walk: "Your praying grandmother, mama, auntie, and cousin 'nem have lives and memories worth keeping alive so that you can run your race. So yes, I invoke the presence and guidance of my ancestors in my daily practice . . . I look to their lives when my faith in God is both tested and tried."[11]

The practice of ancestral veneration can also be the act of adding flesh to the divine, a metaphysical version of the "telephone" game that you may have played as a child. When I commune with my long-deceased grandmother, I don't imagine her waving some wand and granting whatever I desire. She doesn't have that power. But I do picture her knocking on God's door, asking Him to "please sprinkle a little favor on my baby." It's calling in all the love I have at my disposal to make life a little easier to bear. A grandmother's prayers never dissipate.

Examples of ancestral veneration are steeped into our culture. We turn funerals into celebrations of life. We lay flowers on headstones and place cremated ashes on our mantle. We collect family obituaries to maintain knowledge of the family line. All acts of remembering and giving honor to a life that meant something to its people.

Those of us who have lost someone we loved understand the pain that separation causes. At its core, ancestral veneration allows us the healthy space to grieve as we see fit.

Building out the relationship between you and your ancestors allows you to see your role in the bigger picture. It allows you to know that your actions will trickle down into your descendants' lives. We are all connected. We're all working together, trying to figure out how to give life meaning.

It takes some of the pressure off, as you recognize that our time on this planet is finite. The days are long but the years are short. We don't have to get it all right. We don't have to have all the answers or do all the things in order to have a life that's rich and meaningful and beautiful to witness.

We don't have to be perfect to be loved.

RELATIONSHIP WITH NATURE
Finding the Divine in Nature

WHEN I FIRST moved into my house, it had a huge garden plot in the backyard, measuring 12 feet by 12 feet. After we got settled in right at the start of spring, the neighbors told me that the previous owners had been prolific gardeners and had even shared their bounty with the neighborhood. My immediate neighbor told me he loved being able to get tomatoes from right next door.

However, as a 23-year-old with a toddler running around my feet and an infant on my hip, as well as a full-time job, I reassured him that they would have to run to the grocery store for tomatoes from now on because the neighborhood farmer I was not.

But when my life slowed down a bit and my kids went to school full-time, I reassessed my views on plant life. I had managed to keep two children thriving for several years. Why couldn't I keep—at bare minimum—a succulent alive?

I started with one aloe, a plant that would also be useful with its medicinal gel, and named her Bunny, short for Abundance. I then bought three more plants and named them what I wanted to manifest in my own life: Joy, Harmony, and Bliss.

As they grew, I grew.

I discovered that to be a good plant mom, you need to cultivate a life of patience. Having multiple plants requires me to slow down, breathe deep, and focus my attention on the matter at hand. While I'm repotting or misting or analyzing my plants for signs of distress, that's the only thing on my mind. It's one of the purest forms of self-care I know.

Cultivating our spiritual walk within the boundaries of nature calls us back to the beginning. The Christian creation story begins in the Garden, with the earth forming and sprouting all kinds of lush vegetation and varied animal life before humans ever existed.

But the story of the Garden of Eden is not the only one that exists. I've long been drawn to Indigenous creation stories and their depiction of nature as a welcoming, nourishing source of all that is good. In *Braiding Sweetgrass,* botanist Robin Wall Kimmerer, a member of the Citizen Potawatomi Nation, introduces readers to the Skywoman story. In this origin tale, Skywoman emerges from above, falling from Skyworld to a water-logged earth with fruits and seeds from the Tree of Life in her grasp. Animals (geese, swans, beavers, fish, among them) all come to her aid. Finally, a great turtle arrives and offers his shell as ground zero for what we now call North America. Skywoman spreads mud from the bottom of the water onto the shell of the turtle and dances and sings in gratitude. As she praises, what is brown turns green and an abundance of flowers, trees, and other vegetation grows impressively.

In this Indigenous retelling, Skywoman is our "ancestral gardener," Kimmerer writes. A woman is at the center of earth's creation, bringing with her everything we need to survive. These stories remind me how awe-inspiring nature is. Have you ever *really* looked at all the miracles around you? Tiny acorns become oak trees. Seeds buried deep in soil grow their way to the surface, unfurling vines and fruits hundreds of times their original size. Vegetation reaches for the sun across the sky. If you were transplanted on a different planet and saw these same processes, you'd swear it was magic.

When I'm in nature, digging around in the dirt or walking in a local park, I'm reminded that I *am* nature. I'm not an observer; I'm on the main stage. I have a role to play among the trees, the flowers, the grass, the bees. I am part of a much larger framework. My existence matters, even when white supremacy, capitalism, racism, sexism (name your *-ism*) try to convince me otherwise.

Poet Camille T. Dungy considers gardens "centers of resistance."[12] In *Soil: The Story of a Black Mother's Garden,* she documents the multiyear effort to transform her Colorado lawn from a flat, homogenous green space to a lush garden full of native plants, variety as far as the eye can see. Her book is an ode to communal and spiritual growth. "Whether a plot in a yard or pots in a window, every politically engaged person should have a garden," Dungy wrote. "The green of growing things calms me. Plants stabilize me. And I am interested in the patience that is required as I wait for growth. For the politically engaged person—any of us—such patience is a key to survival. Patience is a kindness that carries me through long days and longer nights."

There's something about sticking your fingers in the soil, learning something new, and putting effort into something that will give you a beautiful return. It doesn't always work (my attempt to grow cilantro from seeds has been a failure three years in a row), but it's all data. You learn and adapt for next time.

It's spiritual. It's a safe space. It's calming. It reminds us that just as we are gentle and patient with discovering how to take care of our plants, we need to keep that same energy when it comes to our own care.

Vicky Butler, 70, grew up outside Atlanta with a gang of siblings and a mother who loved to garden. Predictably for those who know mother-daughter dynamics, Butler wasn't interested in following in her mother's footsteps back then. "As a child, in the South, you know how Black mothers are—they make you get out and learn how to do everything. She would make me get out there and dig in the dirt with her and tell me I needed to learn how to do these things. And I hated it."

But about thirty years ago, something shifted. After Butler caught herself admiring neighborhood flowers, her mother's lessons came back full force. She was grateful. "First of all, there's something about being outside in among God's creation and breathing in fresh air. I like getting my hands in that clay, in that soil. I can't explain it other than I feel rejuvenated. I feel energized. It's that sense of new growth and renewal. It just fills my soul and it gives me hope." Butler pauses for a minute. "Yes, it gives me hope."

Like me, Butler began with small houseplants before moving outside. Caring for plants inside the home is a common practice for Black women, an attempt to bring nature's serenity indoors. As I flip through old photo albums, I marvel at how much greenery—spider plants, palms, aloes—I spot in the background of gatherings at my grandmother's house. All this time I figured I didn't have a green thumb. Perhaps I just needed to remember where I came from.

That remembrance fuels Natasha Nicholes, 43, creator of We Sow We Grow, an urban farming nonprofit in Chicago's West Pullman neighborhood. The predominantly Black community has its share of vacant lots and crumbling housing stock, something Nicholes believes can change through the power of plants.

"We wanted to build a community of people who spoke to each other and who looked out for each other," she told me. "The root of the project was to get people to care about each other again. Like they did when I was growing up. And we were using what Black folks often use—food—to connect."

You name it, the lots owned by We Sow We Grow provide it—garlic, squash, greens, onions, tomatoes, and more. Harvest season brings people outside and down the street for fresh food in a long-term food desert. They don't have to go far to get what they need, which is something of a spiritual blessing. Between the bounty of food and the cleanup days the organization hosts, a deeper sense of pride is growing rapidly in their Chicago neighborhood, Nicholes told me.

"I want to feel like we are a part of a community and I want our community to become so strong and to come to the realization that their words and actions and living in this space mattered. And that they would be heard and that we could make a lot of noise and be important. Because for the longest time a lot of the people in the neighborhood that we moved into had not been listened to."

When we chatted, Nicholes was acquiring four more vacant lots in the neighborhood to fill with community-grown produce. The project, nearly a decade in the making, has fulfilled her in the deepest way. When I ask her about this soul work, she visibly lights up.

"That's where getting connected with the Earth helps a lot," she told me. "Because for me, I'm COGIC [Church of God in Christ] born and raised. So the farm has given me a totally different look at my relationship with God and understanding that my ministry doesn't always have to be so staunch. Ministry doesn't always have to happen in church. And ministry doesn't always have to happen with the ability to preach or the ability to slap some blessed oil on somebody. Ministry happens when you meet people where they are and see the humanity in them when nobody else is seeing it."

Amen.

As Nicholes talked, it became clear that it's not just about feeding people and building community, it's also about changing the atmosphere and giving people something to believe in—providing brightness where conditions look bleak.

"I wish that we smiled more," she said simply. "My husband and I have driven around the neighborhood often to see what we need to be paying attention to. And one of the things that I told my husband is that a lot of the folks, they don't look happy. They look beaten down, and they look tired. And they look like they are just sick of the same old, same old. And before I leave this earth, I want to see a difference in the faces."

RELATIONSHIP WITH THE DIVINE
Doing Church Differently

AS A PASTOR, Rev. Courtney Clayton Jenkins of South Euclid, Ohio, implemented virtual service options well before the pandemic, embracing social media in a way that allowed me to follow along with most of her sermons without ever leaving my home.

"People are stretched so thin, that then they don't want to even come to church, they don't have the energy for it," Pastor Jenkins told me. "We get a lot of people who watch at home, but then every once in a while they'll come in, they'll be like, 'Dang, like, I need to be here. I didn't realize how much the physical environment is uplifting to me in a different kind of way.' But then it's just the energy to get up and to make that commitment."

Reverend Jenkins faced her own reckoning with being stretched thin. Her response—an annual July sabbatical—opened new doors for her.

When we spoke, she told me that it is not just a time to reflect and recharge, but it is a cornerstone of her ministry. She is expecting everyone to sabbatical with her and slide into a rhythm of ease during July.

Her 2022 sabbatical, which stretched for sixteen weeks and was funded in part by a grant from the Lilly Foundation, remains the biggest proof that sabbaticals birth great ideas. She traveled to Bali and Indonesia, inviting six friends to join her as she explored how she could lead in a way that felt authentic.

A friend nudged Jenkins to document her travels, so she hired a production assistant to capture the spiritual growth on film. The pastor came back with two short films: *Into the Water,* featuring Jenkins and her six friends in a Balinese water purification ritual, and *Come to the Table,* a dinnertime chat about aging, womanhood, strength, and grief with those same friends. I attended the premiere of both films at a local performing arts theater. Women to my left and right were crying quietly as we listened to the women on-screen share their most vulnerable truths. I marveled at how spiritually fed I felt as I left. It was one of the most honest displays of *goodness* that I'd seen in years. I rarely felt like that after listening to a pastor preach, no matter how solid the message.

"This filmmaking is the future of preaching," she told me between meetings at her church. "Maybe it might just be the future of preaching for me, but I do believe that we need more visual sermons rather than just audible ones. As visual as the upcoming generation is, it's going to be really key in this day and age. I'm able to more intentionally curate those moments through film than I am through my preaching style. That film piece is all divinely inspired, but it is also very much what I think the future of ministry has a possibility of looking like. Because within every congregation there are great stories. And as the pastor, you just have to listen."

This is how we do "church" differently.

UNCONVENTIONAL FELLOWSHIPPING

I'm always on the hunt for spaces to explore my faith in new ways. Unfit Christian Congregation (UCC) was one of the first spaces I encountered that allowed for the totality of who we are, my full humanity. Not just tolerated, but like expected and encouraged. Case in point: I had never seen a "church" where we could talk openly about sex, desire, and sexual orientation, outside of discussions about celibacy. Even the most progressive of churches I've visited still tiptoe around the topics that carry extraordinary resonance in our lives.

UCC founder Danyelle Thomas saw the need to do faith differently, even as her own personal history is steeped in traditional Christianity. "I'm a PK [preacher's kid], so I'm like next level church girl," Thomas told me. "There was really never an option *but* God for me. So where some people come into a relationship with their faith, it is through their own journey. For me, it was just as normal as being Black and being named Danyelle."

As she got older and studied the word, she noticed there were elements to her faith (the way the Black church has demonized the LGBT community, for one) that didn't sit well with her.

"Black churches have a lot of Africanity in our worship and expression, but a lot of white supremacy in our theology," she said. "Not intentionally so, but through a matter of survival, through a matter of inheritance, through all of these things, we end up with a lot of white supremacist theology. And so a lot of the ways in which I saw myself were through the lens of supremacy and not through the eyes of God."

Thomas began writing her musings on Facebook. Thinking nothing of it, she'd post publicly about all things Christianity—celibacy, social justice, Holy Week—with her own clever wordsmithing to draw people in. She had enough of a following to create a Facebook group, and the numbers kept growing. After a few years, she had enough confidence to launch Unfit Christian Congregation. Members meet up offline, a few marriages have popped off, and weekly discussions of pop culture through a spiritual lens keep the comments section jumping.

"I was trying to follow the formula, but what God gave me was a community of people who were ready to do faith differently," Thomas said. "That space formed truly out of organic desire for folks who loved God but could not find themselves within their pews and their fellowship halls and their women's empowerment, brunches and prayer breakfasts and all the things that they had done to seek out community that was familiar to them within those spaces."

We're seeking places where we can breathe and ask the heavy question: *God, what do I need to do to feel your presence?* More and more we're seeing that spiritual fulfillment found in unconventional spaces.

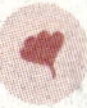

AS WITH MOST things, it was the food that caught my attention first. When a good friend posted that she was brainstorming the menu for her upcoming Bible study series, I stopped what I was doing to weigh in.

Frechic Burton, 39, was following a call that had been placed on her heart for some time. For years, she had been looking for in-person opportunities to connect with people outside of regular church service, but even a few years past the height of the pandemic, most gatherings were still virtual. She decided to create a short-term project to gauge if those in her community felt the same nudge to get up close and personal.

She curated nine different sessions on varied topics—what does the Bible say about dating? About mental health? Parenting? Every other week she invited a few friends and friends-of-friends to join her in her home for a home-cooked meal and spiritual discussion. "We're sitting on the floor, we're on pillows. We're on the couch, we are hanging out. There's kids running around. This is just a very relaxed atmosphere."

Burton envisioned something that was more "Sunday dinner" than "Sunday service," offering soul food favorites like baked chicken, fried cabbage, rice and gravy, and candied yams for guests who make the commitment to come. "I want to make something that is gonna be fresh and wholesome, something that people could look forward to. When we fellowship, especially in our culture, we fellowship with food. It was just very important for me to kind of allow people to let their guard down and not have the intimidation that comes with being within the church walls."

Indeed, most guests who show up at the Bible study attend church regularly but sought a more private space to wrestle with topics near and dear to their heart. For Burton, making her home available for those looking to go deeper in their spiritual walk brings her incredible peace. "One of the things that I remember that the early church did that was very impactful is meeting in people's homes. I always thought that that was so weird. Why would they let people in their house? That seems to be the most intimate place on earth, to be in your house. That's our sacred place. That's not open to the public."

But it's a calling, she affirmed, and she looks forward to seeing what else can happen when you simply invite people in. "A lot of people have trauma associated with being in church. A lot of people are saved but don't know anything about the Bible. I just wanted to get together with everyone and see what does the Bible actually say about all this stuff? And be able to filter it through all our lived experiences."

With four kids (including her 5-month-old son Kendrick, born fifteen years after her next-youngest child), time for herself is at a premium. Her two middle children still live at home (her eldest is off at college), and though they haven't yet joined in, she hopes they take something away from the discussions happening under their own roof. I had to ask her: Girl, why did you decide to make this happen, including making a spread for roughly ten additional people?

"I want Kendrick to be able to grow up seeing me," she said simply. "If someone snaps a photo of him and me on the floor with a Bible in front of us in the living room, surrounded by other people doing the same thing, that's what I want. I never wanna lose the part of me that is ambitious enough to do something like this."

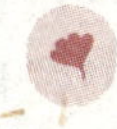

WHEN I SPOKE with my aunt, Reverend Hopkins, whose job is to supervise more than fifty churches in northern Texas, she confirmed my hunch: The future of the church looks less like formal congregations where the pastor preaches every Sunday, but more like people getting together to share their lives in a way that's natural. She shared one example from a church that found a way to do small group gatherings differently—Bark 'n' Bible at a local dog park.

"And people who don't go to church, but love their dogs, bring their dogs," she told me. "The church that she's affiliated with brings the coffee and the donuts. They sit for a little bit and talk about what's happening in their life. And then the associate pastor of the larger church comes and does a ten-minute devotion. And those people go to that thing religiously. And that's what church is becoming."

Even as an ordained reverend who has a fondness for traditional church, she's not wringing her hands over the shift. "Jesus created *communities*," she stressed. "He didn't go somewhere and set up a tent and stay there forever. He created communities. And then empowered others to go out. There's so many things that we have just forgotten. We made church about business, we made church about power, we made church about showmanship. And I can say this because I've been a part of that."

As part of her ministry, she encounters the "Nones and Dones," those folks who aren't tethered to any church and those who don't want to be. Often they feel like they're missing something but they're reluctant to get back in church. Her job is to meet them where they are, my aunt told me, and ensure their spiritual nourishment, no matter what it looks like.

"How are you feeding your soul?" Reverend Hopkins wondered. "You say you're spiritual. Let's talk about where you are. Are you a person that meditates? Are you a person that loves it through music and you play or you listen? Are you an art person? I don't really care what your mode is, but I want your mode to be used repeatedly. You do that and you're connecting with the divine."

TEND TO YOUR SPIRITUAL WELLNESS

FOR THOSE OF us with a complicated relationship with religion, understand that spiritual wellness is less about organized religion and more focused on your own personal relationship with the world around you and your place in it. A few spiritual activities to fill your spiritual cup:

AFFIRMATIONS

Affirmations work by tapping deep into the meat of who you are. Reading and reciting affirmations are proven to have a positive effect on the mind, giving you a better headspace to operate from. Simple affirmations like "I am holy" or "I am part of the fabric of the universe" remind you that you are deserving of good things, always.

NATURE APPRECIATION

Taking a walk might not feel like a spiritual practice but it allows us to be one with creation. Seeing the leaves change, the wind blow, the rain fall . . . all of those connect us to earth and ground us in a way that is holy. My favorite spiritual practice is to sit on the porch and meditate while it rains. Each day, note the weather. Even the rain holds goodness and wonder.

A QUIET PLACE

Give yourself an opportunity to stop moving so much. Quiet allows us to breathe deep, reflect, and get direction. If you don't currently have a corner of your home dedicated to you finding your center, consider this your nudge to create one.

TILLING THE SOIL: SPIRITUAL WELLNESS JOURNALING QUESTIONS

- In what area of your life could you adopt a slower pace?
- What feeds you the most spiritually?
- If you developed your own 10 (or 20!) Commandments, what would they be?
- If you designed your own "church," what would it look like?
- What do you need to release in order to feel your divinity?

Settling Our Nerves

MENTAL AND EMOTIONAL WELLNESS

My great-grandmother was the center of her own world. That is not how women are conditioned. Even now, the family is the center of your world. The children, the relationship, even for independent women, the career is the center, you know? But she was truly the center of her own world. And she loved us and we knew it. And she was able to be there for us without decentering herself, without making us the center. I swear that's why she lived to be 100. Her boundaries were really firm, but they weren't hostile. She would do it in a way where you couldn't get offended. She'd be like, *Oh, no, no. I'm not gonna be able to do that.* But you knew that what she could do, she would do.

—Michelle Smith, 47, poet

EXPLORING THE ROOTS

IN HER MEMOIR, *Bits and Pieces*, Whoopi Goldberg shared the story of her mother Emma Johnson's nervous breakdown, the result of an accumulation of stress as a single mother of two in the Chelsea projects in the 1960s. As an 8-year-old, she came home to watch her mother go into the kitchen, get on her knees, and place her head in the oven. Startled and confused, she ran to get a neighbor, who intervened. Shortly thereafter, her mother was placed in a mental institution. No adults in Goldberg's life explained what was going on. She would not see her mother again for two years.

As dire as it was, her mother's situation was not unheard of or uncommon in our communities. During enslavement, family members and others on the plantation would care for those deemed mentally ill, but mental hospitals were where we first accessed professional mental health services in large numbers.

Founded in 1855, St. Elizabeth's in Washington, DC, was one of the first federally funded mental institutions and the first to accept Black people as patients, a full decade before slavery ended. As you can probably imagine, conditions were less than ideal for Black patients. While the hospital was built on 350 acres (making the property twice as big as Disneyland), lodging for Black and white patients was segregated. Black residents occupied small wooden lodges surrounding the larger center brick building, where white patients received care. Some of these Black residents were soldiers struggling with mental illness exacerbated by war. Others were brought in by family members or police.

A dive into my own family history revealed stints in psychiatric care. My maternal great-grandmother, Minnie Barrett, perhaps buckling under the weight of raising her young children alone after a mob of white men lynched her husband, was institutionalized when my grandmother was a teen. Ancestry records tell me she was a patient at the Ohio State Hospital for Insane for two years. During that time, my grandmother was sent away to live with another family. My mother, having heard the story in bits, tells me my grandmother was deeply affected by her mother's absence. Who wouldn't be?

Our ancestors absolutely knew they were going through stressful and traumatic situations. They absolutely faced impossible scenarios that left their mark on their psyche. They were not and we are not superhuman. Life does indeed leave its mark.

Just because our mothers and grandmothers didn't have a name for their experiences or an expectation that things could be different, it doesn't mean the burden wasn't hard. It doesn't mean they didn't silently wish for better days. It simply means they accepted where they were and did their best to cope with the hand they were dealt, even as it shaped them in ways they couldn't possibly predict or express.

As former *Essence* editor Susan L. Taylor wrote, "Most of our ancestors never spoke about the wrenching pain of losing loved ones, the repeated rapes, the unspeakable acts of violence and humiliation they withstood. But not speaking of the immeasurable harm and how it left them did not make the wounds less deep or the scars less defining. . . . Yes, we are the children of brave survivors, but those survivors did not only pass down to us their courage, they also passed down their pain. We are still in recovery."[1]

I SPENT THREE YEARS talking to elder Black women who spent their younger years running after dozens of kids, maintaining a pristine house, and dealing with the racist hell that awaited them once they stepped outside their doors. Rarely would I hear these women, the Gardeners, express frustration or a wish for a different outcome when recalling these memories.

When I interviewed my paternal grandmother, I got to hear all the details of her life before she was Grandma, from when she was just Alma Louise. At one point, in the 1960s, she moved cross-country to follow my grandfather from Buffalo to San Francisco. By her mid-twenties, she was raising three kids and running an informal in-home daycare in a brand-new city, in a brand-new state. She shook her head when I asked if she felt she needed more support. "I didn't even have time to think about that," she told me matter-of-factly. "I was busy."

I'll admit—sometimes I wish I had her fortitude. If I answer three emails and run two errands on the same day, I'm ready for a nap! These can't be the same genes that helped my foremothers survive the Jim Crow South.

What is the difference between me and my grandmother? Between you and who came before you?

Privilege. Perspective. Time.

That's it.

Our ancestors worked through everything that plagued them because *they had no choice.* We can hold them up as strong women who maintained strength and dignity under indescribable circumstances *and also* acknowledge they deserved better.

Their medicine was their faith and their community, whether it was church, community groups, family, friends. That was what they leaned on when the load got too heavy to bear.

But please believe the load was always heavy.

We are not weak because some of us, in our time, have the privilege of choice. After all, wasn't that the goal? I'd like to imagine my great-grandmother dreamed of a time where her descendants could live and move freely, to tend to themselves without fear or punishment. Our ancestors deserved that privilege of resting when they were tired or space to mourn when they suffered a loss. My wake-up call at 26, where a doctor looked me up and down and gave me a literal prescription to rest, probably saved my life. I had the ability and the privilege to choose something else for myself, to walk away from job commitments that were increasing my stress levels and accelerating my aging. I had the opportunity to choose me. Our ancestors deserved that opportunity as well.

This chapter is about what we know now that perhaps our ancestors didn't know then—yes, "stressed" is a state of mind but it is also a series of internal processes that happens without much input from us at all. Stressors come and go, that's for sure, but the effects of that stress will linger, particularly if we are accumulating stress without moving it through our mind and body.

As humans, we are divinely engineered to survive. When our brains encounter something that we (either consciously or unconsciously) perceive as a threat, we have hormones within our body that help us respond—adrenaline is one of them. After the threat has passed, other chemicals swoop in to help us calm down and get back to our baseline.

More formally, this is the autonomic nervous system in action.

It has a few branches that help us navigate troubled waters: the sympathetic nervous system, which controls our "fight or flight" response, and the parasympathetic nervous system, which gets us back to chill mode.

This is a good system! Envision it as a friend who hypes you up before a big presentation at work and another friend who takes you out to get a massage afterward. But for some of us, our sympathetic nervous system is on overdrive—not just hyping us up but making us ask hard questions: *What if this doesn't go well? Will I get fired? How will I pay my bills?* For those folks, they are living most of their lives stuck in fight or flight.

Therapist and author Jennifer Sterling always says the opposite of depression isn't happiness—it's vitality. It's feeling alive in your body, something that can't often happen when you are stuck in fight or flight or a dysregulated nervous system. This chapter is about shifting our minds and bodies out of chaos and into a state of calm and vitality, as best we can.

The bottom line is Black women are underresourced when it comes to mental and emotional care, but we're eager to do what we can to fill the gap. We're reading books, devouring podcasts, engaging with friends, and leaning into the spaces where we can be ourselves most authentically. We're trying our best to heal in a society that makes it a full-time job. We're doing the work and hoping others will meet us halfway.

Let me say this up front: I'm a researcher and journalist who has spent the last ten years knee deep in the practices Black women have depended on to be mentally and emotionally well. What we're doing in this chapter is walking through life together, helping you sort through the chronic stressors in your life that are contributing to or worsening your mental and emotional health.

There's not much we can do about those random, everyday stressors. Your alarm didn't go off so you're late for work. You stubbed your toe on the edge of the bed and it throbs the rest of the day. You got an email that your daughter didn't turn in her homework assignment. You get the idea.

But chronic stress? Chronic stressors are where we can actually shift the weight of what ails us. The problem with chronic stress is we may not even recognize what these chronic stressors are. They're just the hum in the background. In this chapter we're identifying the best strategies for mental and emotional well-being, while also investigating some hidden stressors and how to lessen their impact on your life. Together let's figure out how to be mentally and emotionally well with all the tools at our disposal.

WHO TAUGHT YOU ABOUT MENTAL/ EMOTIONAL WELL-BEING?

I DIDN'T HAVE the language for it then but in hindsight it's clear: In elementary school, I was an anxious mess. The days where I had to speak in front of the class were the worst. I'd wake up with a churning stomach, sweat beading on the forehead, arms shaky. On particularly bad days, I'd have to vomit before I'd be able to speak.

One of my most vivid memories was sitting in the backseat of my parents' car before school and calming myself down by mentally walking myself through the entire day, ending with dinner, the highlight.

What was going on that day? Nothing noteworthy I can remember.

Anxiety has always been my baseline. The feeling that *something somewhere was wrong* followed me from childhood to my present reality as a mother of two in my thirties. I didn't know what was wrong or how to express it. This is just how I'm built, I figured.

But even as the anxiety became a close friend, I also managed to find a few lessons on calm and better mental health as a student at a Catholic all-girls high school. (I don't know how my parents managed to afford tuition for myself and my two sisters, but we all had a private school education.)

My theology teacher, Jeannette DeCorpo, was the first "hippie" I had ever met. She wore Birkenstocks and was deeply in love with her dog Latte. For the early 2000s, she was remarkably progressive. She taught lessons on sexuality and inclusion and urged us to give great care to our classmates who might be struggling mentally.

On several occasions, she would conduct our class in the chapel, instead of in our regular classroom. We would each find a comfortable spot to lie down on the floors or in the pews. We'd use our book bags as pillows and put our sweaters over our eyes and we'd breathe softly as she played instrumental meditation music.

I can't speak for my classmates, but I'd be knocked out for forty minutes. A few minutes before the bell would ring, she'd softly urge us to get up, take some deep breaths, and be ready to go to our next class.

She was teaching us *the power of a pause*. We were children, yes, but we were balancing a lot—challenging schoolwork, extracurriculars, jobs, friendships. There was a lot of pressure on our young shoulders, and I appreciate that she took a minute to recognize it.

In exchange for that hefty tuition check was exposure to different ways of thinking and being. Administrators at my school were determined to build sisterhood among the student body, and every other week we would have some type of assembly or gathering to celebrate each other. We had yearly retreats, a staple of which were our affirmation letters, where friends would write pages and pages of how much they valued having you in their life. It was perhaps the best investment my parents could have given me—the opportunity to be steeped in this real-world vision of what wellness could look like.

WHO TAUGHT YOU ABOUT MENTAL/EMOTIONAL WELLNESS?

- As a child, were you able to express how you felt or was that considered "talking back"?
- Was there a divide between children's problems and adult problems?
- Did anyone in your family ever attend any type of therapy session?
- Do you recall any conversation about a family member's mental troubles, whether cloaked in euphemism or stated plainly?
- Have you ever been told by adults to "fix your face" or otherwise conceal your true feelings?
- What were you taught about mental/emotional health? Where did the women in your family put their worries, their stress, their mental illness?

WHY ARE BLACK WOMEN SO DAMN STRESSED ALL THE TIME?

MY LEAST FAVORITE online skits are the ones mocking Black moms. Often it's a young Black man in a bonnet and robe with a leather belt, threatening "her" imaginary kids for some minor infraction, like forgetting to take the meat out of the freezer for dinner or daring to ask for a toy at the store. We're often portrayed as loud, abrasive, and quick to dole out punishment.

I've always looked at those skits with a critical eye. (I am very fun at parties.) As I scrolled through the comments, I wondered why these portrayals hit home for so many. Why did everybody seemingly grow up with a quick-tempered mom?

What is more likely (and what research suggests) is that Black women are undersupported. The majority of Black women I know are being asked to shoulder more than any one person should—they have to raise children, be outstanding employees, "submit" to their partners, praise and worship, be a role model, take care of home, eat healthily, sweat four times per week, keep their hair nice, be politically active, find time to have a good orgasm or two, and be involved in the community. Oh, and do all that while navigating racism and sexism.

So, yes, it then becomes a big deal that the chicken is still frozen when they get home at six. Where is our help?

What people perceive as "attitude" is usually exhaustion. But we knew that, didn't we? A Black woman doesn't typically say, "I'm depressed." Instead it'll sound like, "I'm tired." Our depressive symptoms tend to be somatic—we feel it in the body before we express it verbally.[2] This means our struggles often go underreported in spaces where we need to count most—in our homes, physicians' offices, and in scientific data.

And even when we do express our fatigue and overwhelm, we are often encouraged to keep pressing on anyway. Recently, my niece, a beautiful 20-something single mom of two young kids, posted on social media that she was tired and on the brink of quitting nursing school due to the pressure of single-handedly keeping all these separate balls in the air. All the comments?

"You got this!"

"Keep going!"

"Don't you dare quit!"

Her friends and family were all well-meaning but damn, she just said she was struggling. Can she get some *help*? Often we confuse encouragement with support. Is anyone offering to watch her children for an afternoon so she can study in peace?

This is the conundrum of the Strong Black Woman archetype. Because we *do* the impossible, people think we can do the impossible.

During one period where my anxiety was horribly out of control, my husband gifted me a copy of Dr. Angela Neal-Barnett's *Soothe Your Nerves,* the first book on psychology written by a Black woman I had ever read. It was a good reminder that even though we haven't always been able to name what's weighing us down, those weights have been there. Dr. Neal-Barnett conducted a study of self-identified "Strong Black Women," asking them to track their daily activities in a diary while tracking physical stress markers such as blood pressure and heart rate.

What struck the researcher most was the incongruity between how the respondents described their days versus what their blood pressure and heart rate data was reporting. They would report in their diaries that the day was "calm," but their blood pressure and heart rate spiked in time with events the researchers would consider stressors. In one instance, a participant reported no real stress had occurred, but as Dr. Neal-Barnett reviewed her activity diary, she saw the participant had fired a member of her team that same day and during that period, her blood pressure spiked 30 percent. After the interview portion of the study, the doctor realized the women knew they were stressed but were choosing not to dwell on or name it. "I wouldn't be able to get anything done if I was worrying about how I felt," one said.

The strength and perseverance we exude is born out of necessity. In spaces where we are not protected, we protect ourselves. This armor is heavy and we've built up the muscle to be able to carry it well.

By the time I take my last breath, I want to know that I did my part to coax Black women to give less of a damn about holding up the world at all costs and instead devote themselves to the courageous work of being completely, unapologetically human.

WHERE DO YOU GO WHEN THINGS GET TOO HEAVY?

SITTING IN THE therapist's waiting room, waiting for the first of three free appointments courtesy of my job's employee assistance program, my stomach was churning. *Had I really done it?*

The therapist was a middle-aged, heavyset white woman with long, frizzy blond hair that looked like it was on its way to turning gray. She poked her head out into the waiting room and called my name. I gathered my items and followed her into the privacy of her office.

"Well, what brings you in today?" She flipped open her notebook, her pen poised above the paper, eyes looking at me expectantly.

"I'm . . ." I struggled to find the words. *Why was I there? What was I hoping to fix?*

At the time I was a 24-year-old wife and mother to two children under 4, an overwhelmed grad student and full-time nonprofit employee with a hellish commute. Even four years into motherhood, I hadn't found my stride or a place to catch my breath. I hadn't yet come to terms with what motherhood was doing to my life, expanding and constricting it at the same time. Handling all of this at 24 also had me coping with a long-simmering resentment of how my life choices had rocketed me past my peers (and husband, quite honestly) in terms of mindset and responsibility. I felt like I needed a safe space to sort all this out, to do something about the mental fatigue and exhaustion I was battling through every day. I had picked up the phone, made the appointment and the twenty-five-minute drive in the hopes that this therapy journey would be the first step to a better, more content, more well-rested me.

After I explained all that to the therapist, she nodded and scribbled in her notebook.

Her next question: "Well, are you on birth control now? Have you got that under control?"

I can't quite remember my answer to her, but I stammered out something in the affirmative. I kept replaying that question in my head. *Would she have asked a white woman that? Why jump to my ability to have more children instead of, I don't know, learning more about my life and the context that I was presenting? What if I wasn't on birth control? What then? Would she have lectured me about not being responsible?*

Without realizing it, a wall went up. We chatted politely for the rest of the session and that was that. I kept the second appointment to see if my initial hunch was wrong, but it wasn't. We weren't a good match.

I share this memory because it's crucial to understand that therapy, like many tools we may use to strengthen our mental and emotional health, is not a one-and-done process. It takes time, investment, energy, and patience to find the right avenue that works for you.

While that may feel deflating, understanding that the process is a journey will allow you to withstand the ebbs and flows rather than expect you will find a miracle your first time at bat. I know how hard it is to show up to that first therapy session. You wonder: *Can I afford this? Is this situation bad enough? Can I handle it myself? Can I tell a stranger my true feelings? What will they say about me?*

Especially as a Black woman seeking a Black therapist within your network, which can make the process one long waiting game. Only 5 percent of the US psychology workforce is Black.[3] Slots get filled faster than Black women can get credentialed.

Matching yourself with a Black female therapist is simply a matter of numbers, availability, and location. With the numbers being low as they are, you may not be able to find a Black therapist your first time, even using an online directory as a guide. Cultural competency should be top of your list, but a therapist who specializes in your area of need is worth their weight in gold.

This may be controversial, but I'll say it anyway: Maybe your *aha!* moment won't come from a spot on a couch across from a woman of the same hue.

Hear me out!

A couple months after my first attempt I found a new therapist, also white, but closer in age and location. She was short and Southern and reminded me a bit of actress Ellie Kemper—red hair and a smiley face. During our first session, she asked the same question, a common part of the intake process: "What brings you in today?"

After I gave her my whole life history (I am physically incapable of telling a "long story short"), she nodded thoughtfully and asked the question somebody should have asked me years ago: "And in what way would support from your family, friends, community help you with those goals?"

I was stunned. She was urging me to reframe my life from a solitary point of view to a communal one, one where I wasn't solely carrying every aspect of my healing.

In its best form, this is what therapy does. It drives home the point that you are worthy, that you matter, that you deserve a safe, comforting space to hash out whatever is preventing you from living life more fully.

Over time, I could feel the fog start to lift. We went from weekly sessions, to every two weeks, to monthly as I progressed. We talked about my week, about situations I'm struggling with, about the areas in my life where I'd like to see improvement. We talked about my strengths, my victories. We talked about the people who have shaped me and the woman I would like to be in the future.

Do I believe that everyone should go to therapy? Quite simply, yes. At least occasionally. Not just any therapist, but a *good* therapist. In the same way I believe everyone should go to the doctor, and some of us must go more than others. Most of us are walking around with issues that would be helpful to lay at the feet of a (good) mental health professional. We can seek support for anger issues, perfectionism, people-pleasing, workplace woes. The list is long.

What (good) therapy has done for me is given me permission to be me, unapologetically. I've found that even if I'm not in "crisis," having a sacred space for me to be wholly myself, free from distractions or obligations, keeps me balanced and in tune with myself, rather than managing everything entirely on my own. The load was too heavy to carry. Therapy gave me a few extra hands.

My therapist worked with me to stop rushing past uncomfortable emotions. For example, I had a tendency to say, "[sad/frustrating thing here] . . . but it's fine." I didn't even realize I was doing that until I brushed something off that I was really struggling with in one of our sessions. She looked me in my eyes and said, "I can see the pain on your face." Dear reader, let me tell you *I broke*. That mask ("Everything is fine!") is so hard to resist. She helped me come to terms with the fact that I don't always have to be the one who radiates strength and energy and solutions to everyone else.

BATTLING STIGMA

AS YOU READ at the beginning of this chapter, Black folks seeking help for their mental troubles isn't new or groundbreaking. When there has been a worthwhile option, we've sought it out, even if it paled in comparison to what our [white] counterparts received or what we truly needed.

The oft-cited stigma of therapy or other mental health interventions, unfortunately, is well-earned. The stigma is actually white supremacy doing the work for us. In the late 1800s, psychologists saw an increase in the number of African Americans presenting with mental health issues. Racial biases being what they were at the time, medical professionals argued we were having a hard time coping with our newfound freedom. They suggested we didn't struggle mentally before because during enslavement, all of our "needs" were taken care of—food, shelter, purposeful work. What would we have been stressed about? Never mind that enslavers certainly didn't care about whether their enslaved populations were mentally fit to work. It was like worrying whether your vacuum was happy. Today the medical establishment has worked to right these previous wrongs, dedicating resources to encourage Black people to not only engage with mental health professionals but join their ranks.[4]

The stigma of therapy almost caused me to miss out on a wonderful blessing. If you admit to the wrong people that you're struggling and you don't think you can manage your mental health alone, they'll come up with a million reasons why you don't need help.

"But you have a great life! What could be wrong with you?"

"You just need to pray. Have you talked to a pastor?"

"Everybody's stressed. What makes you think you're so special?"

"It will pass. You're just in a busy season of life right now."

I've heard all these things and more in discussing my desire to go to therapy. Because of the stigma, when I first started going to therapy all I would tell people is that I "had a doctor's appointment." In doing so I worried my daughter half to death because she thought something was wrong since I was going to the doctor twice a month! After that, I decided then to just be honest. I know therapy is a major reason I feel so much lighter today. Therapy is what got me through some of the hardest parts of my life. And I'm not ashamed to say it.

I met video producer Angelique Dyer, 32, online, as fellow Beyoncé fans and women in media tend to gravitate toward each other. She would post about her anxiety on the same days mine would be flaring quietly. I found her openness refreshing. *We could just . . . talk about what was bothering us? With everybody? Even strangers? Mind blown.*

But when we sat down to talk, she was quick to tell me she wasn't always publicly vulnerable. A turning point for Dyer came during a college study-abroad trip with a diabetic friend. "When we first noticed that we were sparking a friendship, she said, 'I want to let you know that I am diabetic. And I want you to know this in case something happens to me.' She told me, 'I make it a point to tell people that, because I don't want you to panic if something happens to me.' Sure enough, we were sitting in a café where we were living and she had an episode."

Because of her friend's advice, Dyer knew exactly what to do. She got her some orange juice and before long, her friend was back to her normal self.

"It was at that moment I realized it's important to tell the people around you what is going on with you so that they can help you in those moments when you can't help yourself," she told me. "That's when I decided to treat my disorder like something that I'm going to have for the rest of my life. It's not going away. I don't ever see it going away unless I get a new brain that functions differently. And I hear lobotomies are very expensive and I don't really have the time for it."

All jokes aside, Dyer recognized that she had to take control of the narrative she was telling herself. She decided anxiety was nothing to be ashamed of.

"I realized that me being closed off about it, wasn't helping anyone," Dyer said. "It definitely wasn't helping myself because me being closed off to it, felt a bit like shame. It took me a minute to get over that and realize all of the good parts of me are also rooted in my anxiety. And so I stopped seeing it as a shameful thing and started seeing it sort of as my superpower."

Dyer's powers include giving great pep talks ("I have to give myself one every day"), being an outstanding listener, and having an outsized sense of empathy. Another benefit? She is stellar at her job. "I don't think I'd be the producer that I am, if I didn't have an anxiety disorder. I'm able to literally look at every side of everything, every worst-case scenario of what could go wrong. I see that as a great thing. I'm a premortem and postmortem kind of girl. I'm covering all the bases."

In chatting with the youngest Gardener, my 19-year-old niece Janay Jefferson, I appreciated there was a welcome generational shift in the mental health conversation. Less hiding, more openness. Everyone's battling something, they figure, so why be judgy about it?

"A lot of people say our generation is more sensitive," Jefferson said. "But I think it is just that they're more aware of what's going on with others and more sympathetic about what's happening in other people's lives and understanding that that can stop them from performing at their best."

Before you can be open with anyone else, you have to be open with yourself. Ask: *Have I accepted how my brain works and what's going on internally?* Releasing the shame and accepting reality is the first step to erasing the stigma. Stigma can't exist where acceptance resides.

FEELING YOUR FEELINGS: SOMATIC STRATEGIES

AFTER SEVERAL YEARS doing deep work with different therapists, I found myself moving through my life with relative ease. I say "relative" because life continued to throw uppercuts, but the difference was that I could view those obstacles with confidence. A year into the pandemic, however, that confidence was running low, so I booked a session with a new therapist, this time one who had just entered the profession a year or two prior.

A few sessions in, I realized not only was I doing much of the talking, she didn't have much to say that I hadn't already said. I didn't need affirmation at that point, I needed help moving these heavy emotions. I felt like I was drowning and she was on the shore nodding that, *Yes, the waves did seem high today.*

Turns out, this time I didn't need to *talk* about my emotions. I needed to sit with them. Feel them. And then, they would find their way through.

The more I research trauma, emotional regulation, and release, the more I'm convinced God designed the body with such precision. Somatic approaches tap into the body's innate healing power, soothing our nervous system and giving our bodies the sense of calm they've been longing for.

For some of us, traditional talk therapy might be too intense or too uncomfortable. With more somatic modalities, we can tap into our body and therefore soothe the mind.

Before I talk about a couple of somatic approaches, we have to start with the basics—feeling our feelings.

Tara, I'd rather walk backward into oncoming traffic, I hear you saying.

Until recently, I would have said, "Me too."

Sitting with our feelings is uncomfortable. That anxiety/fear/grief/anger that sits in your body and makes it hard for you to speak your mind? We have to acknowledge them and understand their presence.

We have to feel the anxiety in our throat and chest.

We have to feel the sadness in our head making everything heavy and cloudy.

We have to feel the overwhelm in our stomach.

Can I tell you a secret? These emotions that we're running from—they're neutral. They may not *feel* neutral, but they are. There is no hierarchy in which joy reigns supreme at the top and anger, fear, and sadness linger at the bottom. They all coexist and give your internal world color and direction.

But if you can't yet conceptualize "neutral emotions," understand that those feelings are still there even if we don't deal with them. It's like pretending you're not sick even though you have a 104-degree fever and body aches. Ignoring the symptoms doesn't mean you're healthy.

Some of this begins in childhood, Kansas City–based trauma therapist Nadirah Habeebullah told me. "You learn over time that like, *Oh, people don't really like when I speak up or when I ask for what I need, or when I share my emotions and I don't feel very accepted in the family.* As a child, you absolutely have to feel accepted by your caretakers because you can't just go and find another family. You can't just go and get your own house. If the messaging I'm getting is that you gotta stop doing all that because you're doing too much . . . then absolutely a hundred percent I'm going to learn to silence that, not listen to it. But then we grow up, when we leave that environment, we don't live with our parents anymore, but we still carry that same behavior."

If that is your story, don't fret.

"What we have to do now is update those parts of ourselves so that we can realize like, oh, like I'm actually grown now," Habeebullah said. "I actually have a job and I can choose the people that I invite into my life, and I am responsible for myself, for my feelings, and other people are responsible for themselves and their feelings. And even if they don't like the things that I say and that I do, that's okay. And they can deal with that and they can manage that. If our relationship is a strong enough one, we can work through that."

Several Gardeners told me even as adults, they struggle with letting their emotions come to the surface. For Olivia Lauer, a 35-year-old mother of two, accepting and sitting with her own feelings became a gift she gave herself because she knew she needed it.

"I started to validate my own feelings," Lauer said. "I started to give myself the things that I knew no one else was going to give me. Even my family. No one knew what to even say. Because it was always, *well, why do you have an attitude? What's wrong?* Like you're choosing to feel these negative emotions rather than even acknowledging you *should* feel that way, because what happened was really awful. Those conversations didn't happen for any of us from any of our families, because it didn't happen for them."

Still, Lauer maintained a sense of empathy for her family members, especially her mother, through our conversation. "This is where my mother and I differ because I allow myself to sit in my anger and my sadness as to where she doesn't want it to lead to depression and she doesn't want it to manifest into other things," Lauer explained. "Definitely in my early twenties, we had a lot of hard conversations where I just was missing that, but looking back, and even then, I knew she just wanted me to be okay."

We often resist our feelings because if we sit with them, it makes them real and then what will we do? We're ill-equipped for their presence. It's kind of like having rowdy houseguests. You're not sure what kind of damage they will do to your home and if they will leave when asked. It seems counterintuitive to invite them in to have a seat on your couch. But that's precisely what we have to do if we want to become more emotionally fluent.

Recently, when my feelings feel overwhelming, I sit in front of the mirror and look myself in the eye. "You're having some big feelings," I say softly, as if I'm talking to 5-year-old Me. "That's okay. I can handle your big feelings. Let it out."

I do all the things that allow the emotion to come to the surface and stay there. I may scream. I may hum. I hold my hand over my heart and feel the heat rise. I close my eyes and breathe deeply. I go for a walk and mentally visualize the stress leaving my body with each step. I accept the hardest truths, my deepest fears, and I sit with them. It's uncomfortable, for sure, and I'd much rather skip all this shit and just fast-forward to the part where I feel better.

But now I recognize my emotions aren't torturing me. They're meant for reflection. And growth. A reminder that sometimes we can't move forward until we accept where we are.

We go inward.

We sit with ourselves. We lean on those who love us. We feed ourselves. We listen. We learn. We breathe deep.

And sometimes we cry. That release connects us to our body, even in those times when we don't know where those tears are coming from.

"Culturally, as women . . . crying is considered weak, and I disagree," actress Tracee Ellis Ross told *Interview* magazine.[5] "For people and women who have big lives, filled with responsibilities and dreams and all of it, it's important to allow those spaces and times when we've got to cry, whether it's out of gratitude, out of discomfort, or out of grief. But once they start flowing, I think to myself, 'I really needed this.' I'm grateful for them when they come because I think there's a lot of wisdom in them. Like, your body is not lying. My body is often so much wiser than my mind."

We *feel* our way through it.

We need to feel all the emotions, even the ones we don't feel comfortable holding. It's amazing how many Black women I know hold back their anger, sadness, fear, even as we get labeled as aggressive despite our restraint. Professor Brittney Cooper titled her third book *Eloquent Rage* after a student told her she admired how Cooper embodied the principle.[6]

"It feels really important to me to say to Black women that it is okay to be angry," Cooper told NPR. "And it is okay to reclaim that anger because part of what I think then happens is that when we feel the right to be angry, then we also give ourselves the permission to feel any of the other things that we feel in relationship to that anger. And so it is trying to restore intact a sort of full sense of our emotional lives."

Let them all in: Anger is a signal that something is unfair. Sadness is a sign we have lost something we held dear. Grief is love without form. Regret is our internal guidepost showing us the way home. Shame is internalized negative self-evaluation.

Tapping into that rich emotional inner world is the heartbeat of somatic strategies, of feeling and processing what is living in your body.

EMDR (Eye Movement Desensitization and Reprocessing) was my first somatic experience that opened my eyes to many modalities of therapy.

When I first arrived at my therapist's office (a Black woman! Finally!), I expected to meet twice a month and allow her to function as a guide while I talked through some of my issues with self-worth, past trauma, and this ever-increasing anxiety.

And for the first few sessions, that's exactly what we did. She surprised me, however, when she suggested we try EMDR. I was vaguely familiar with the modality, but thought: *Wasn't this for people with more severe trauma?*

In layman's terms, EMDR is a multiphase treatment. During the session, you focus on your core beliefs around distressing moments in your past, and with each session, allow your mind's natural healing response to take place. In some cases you will follow the therapist's finger back and forth; in other cases, they may use alternating hand buzzers, or some other bilateral stimulation. "Resourcing," an invitation to call forth people, places, and situations that feel safe and calm, is often used. As you move through the phases, the distressing event is no longer such a powerful emotional trigger.

During my first session I cried, the release of nearly a decade of tension. As I walked to my car, I could literally feel my body sink into such a state of relaxation that I was disoriented.

To be so "light" was foreign to me. When I went home, I told my husband it felt like I took off a fifty-pound vest.

Four sessions of what I now lovingly call "bad bitch brainwashing" turned me into a believer. Here's the best way I can describe how the EMDR process helped me: Imagine you're in the kitchen and you drop a stack of dishes. There are little shards all over the floor—some you can see, some you can't. But you don't have access to a broom or a tool to help you get them up so you just do your best to navigate around the pieces.

EMDR felt like someone handed me a broom. I could finally sweep all the pieces together into piles. There is more room to function. I can breathe.

Somatic approaches work by reconnecting us to our bodies, reminding us that we can find calm and safety there. Other somatic modalities, like dance therapy, couple movement with healing. If we can move through what is stuck, we can find lightness we previously thought impossible.

If nothing else, we can connect with our breath, the most basic form of somatic work that's always accessible.

Right now, as you're reading, do me a favor:

Close your eyes and take a deep breath. Inhale for four seconds, exhale for four seconds. Do it again. Breathe.

When you feel life getting too busy, too chaotic, too stressful, take a deep cleansing breath. And even when life appears to be sailing along smoothly, pay attention to your breath. Are you holding your breath? Are you breathing too fast?

This, in so many words, is a somatic approach to healing. Our bodies hold grief, sadness, anger, trauma. They also hold joy, peace, and calm in equal measure—if we can tap into it.

REST + REINFORCEMENTS

WHEN I WAS a child, my mother would allow us to take one "personal day" per semester. It was one day where we could tell her that we needed a day to catch up on rest or just not spend all day staring at our teacher.

I didn't think much of it at the time but looking back, my mom was doing some revolutionary parenting. She was teaching us, in her own way, that life can be stressful, and even as children, we had the right to say that we were overwhelmed and could use a break.

I'm thankful for her example because now as an adult and a parent myself, mental health days are the backbone of my rest practice. Those mental health days (or as my bestie calls them, Tara Appreciation Days) are for recognizing when I have been giving more than I have been receiving and doing what I can to restore that balance.

You may have been hearing lots of conversation about rest—much of it attributed to Tricia Hersey, founder of The Nap Ministry. For years she has led the charge for Black women to reconsider the ways they approach "grind culture" and resist capitalism. I owe so much of my own philosophies to her insistence that "We will rest."

We absolutely need to be encouraged to rest. But what is rest without reinforcements? I believe that's the second half of the equation. Someone who is not accustomed to rest is unlikely to put down her to-do list in order to tend to herself. In every conversation or interview I've had with a friend or Gardener, there is a resistance to letting things go undone. Even when I know better, there's still occasions when I push myself a bit too hard and need to be redirected toward rest and care.

Quick story: As I was finishing this book, my husband knew I had been pulling long hours to get to the finish line. He saw me up early one day and encouraged me to go back to sleep. "You're tired," he said. "I can see it on your face."

I'm sure my husband doesn't mind me using him as an example here. But I woke up and hopped out of bed, despite my exhaustion, because I had things to do. In this case, it's easy to tell someone to go lie down, but what can you do that makes that possible? Along with my husband's care and concern (which I greatly appreciate), some tangible support needs to be offered. When he asked what I needed, I told him I needed him to make dinner. Every night. I didn't even want to think about it. Dinner, for me, is tough because it's an hour or two of concentration at the end of an already long day. Taking that off my plate would make it easier for me to rest.

For two months, he handled every part of the dinner process—taking the protein out to thaw, coming up with meal plans, ensuring our daughter with multiple food allergies had her separate meal. And the cherry on top? He handled dishes too. It was the type of support that let my mind breathe and I could rest or write without worrying that I needed to participate in some part of the dinner process.

Rest is crucial, and I've learned that reinforcements make it easier. I'm encouraging you to think about what type of reinforcements you can develop. A common refrain is "I don't know how to rest"—you *do* know how to rest. You're just stuck in the wrong environment. So let's start there. What needs to happen so you can get the rest you need? Who or what can support you in this quest?

SOME COMMON REINFORCEMENTS

A change of scenery—Are you the type of person who can't relax if there's dishes in the sink or laundry to be done? It's a good guess that changing your environment—either retreating to a space where chores are out of your eyeline or leaving that space altogether—will allow you the breathing room you need to rest.

Material support/delegation—Much like my husband and the dinner request, having someone take something off your plate gives you the bandwidth to think about yourself. What could you delete from your to-do list?

Silence—Sensory overload can cause your stress levels to rise without even realizing it. If all else fails, headphones.

Money—Let's be real. More money means more access to resources that make it easier to find time in your day—housekeepers, babysitters, nannies, grocery delivery. Do you need to start a "Treat Yourself" fund, saving each month so you can spend money in ways that help you have breathing room?

Timeline extension—Looming deadlines make it hard to find time to relax, especially if you've been trained with the mindset that you can relax *after* the project is done. While that's often true, pushing yourself in the midst of a stressful project can sometimes backfire, causing you to spin your wheels. An extension could be the thing that opens up the floodgates of creativity to get you to the finish line faster.

Reassurance—In the case of my husband noticing my fatigue, it did do my heart good to hear someone else say what I did not: *You look tired. You should rest.* Perhaps you're the type who needs to hear it's okay. If so, there's nothing wrong with asking for reassurance.

LET'S TALK ABOUT IT: MENTAL HEALTH IN RELATIONSHIPS

WHEN OUR CLOSEST relationships are in a state of consistent upheaval or chaos, it *will* imprint on our psyche. In *Nobody Knows the Trouble I've Seen*, clinical psychologist Dr. Inger Burnett-Zeigler wrote about her hot-and-cold relationship with "Nathan," a partner whose initial charm and generosity drew her in. Before long, she realized all was not well with their love. His mood swings were intense and triggering. After arguments, he would disappear or give her the silent treatment to express his disapproval. She soon found herself overwhelmed in the dysfunctional relationship. "The hyperventilating, thumping heartbeat of anxiety and the heavy well of despair were in an intricate dance, and who was in the lead depended on the day," she admitted.[7] The stress of the relationship led her to therapy for the first time. There, she realized she was in an emotionally abusive relationship. It took years for her to extricate herself from the relationship and find healing.

As I write this, I am in my late thirties. Anecdotally, a lot of my friends' marriages are imploding. As we have moved down the line from idealistic 20-somethings to more seasoned 30-somethings, I've witnessed an uptick in the number of women in my immediate circle who have decided to walk away, no matter what it costs. The threat to their mental health is too great.

I didn't write this section to nudge you out the door, but I do hope it encourages you to consider what your relationship means for your mental health. Whether that's drawing stronger boundaries, changing your own response in the relationship pattern, or giving yourself some space to figure out the best path forward, something needs to change *if something needs to change.*

It takes tremendous energy to be at odds with the person you see most often. And when we lack the tools, skills, or desire to move us from a place of frustration to peace, we languish. We can drink green juices and go to the gym and pray and meditate, but if your romantic partner is not a safe space for you to exhale and be yourself, you are enduring for the sake of enduring. Your mental and emotional health is at risk.

Dawn Rivers, 54, knew her eighteen-year marriage was over in the first year. Their relationship was volatile and explosive before they even made it to marriage. Rivers had even decided to say "no" at the altar but had a last-minute change of heart. The first year, typically a learning curve for most newlyweds, had her ready to throw in the towel. "The church is like, just pray, be a submissive wife, do all the things. And I was like, but should it be this bad? Should I be this unhappy?"

Her husband, a firefighter who struggled with anger and alcohol issues, would lie about everything, big and small. Their arguments kept escalating. Eventually things turned physical. Her desire to stay together for the kids had been replaced by a desire to find peace. Turns out, everybody else wanted peace too. "The summer that I decided that I was going to divorce, I sat our son and our daughter down and I said, your dad and I are getting a divorce. And our daughter said, 'Well, of course. He's never here anyway.'"

Her kids' quick acceptance led Rivers to move forward with the divorce. After eighteen months, she was free. "I was a school librarian. He was a firefighter. People thought, *you guys are the Huxtables.* Y'all got a big tree in the front yard, you got a dog and two kids, you got a house. It's shiny on the outside. It's black on the inside. It is dark up in here and it's broken for what? To stay. For what?"

In conversations with women like Rivers, it's clear we enter relationships with the best of intentions. No one wants to believe they will divorce before the ink is dry or be tangled in the same arguments for the next twenty years.

But relationships are tricky. We can't always predict the ways they grow and shift. Or the ways *we* grow and shift. You often won't know who you are or what you require until you're already coupled. Relationships require a level of vulnerability and communication that most of us will only get within the confines of that pairing. We often enter relationships lacking the skills we need to communicate effectively, negotiate our needs, and show up fully for our partners.

To know whether our relationship is unhealthy, we must circle back to what love actually *is*. In *All About Love*, bell hooks told us: "To truly love we must learn to mix various ingredients—care, affection, recognition, respect, commitment and trust, as well as honest and open communication."[8]

Together, those ingredients feel like home, equaling emotional and psychological safety.

Do you feel like you are home?

When a good friend of mine was teetering back and forth on whether to leave her husband, she'd muse about finding a better fit somewhere, someone who understood her instinctually and wouldn't require so much daily effort to get even the little things right. When she asked me whether she should stay or go, I hesitated because I truly didn't know either. (I also make it a point to support my friends in *their* decisions. My opinion isn't the most important one in the equation.)

My gut, however, told me that the question she was really asking was "Is it bad enough to leave?"

The moment you start asking if it's *bad enough*, you likely have sufficient evidence that the relationship is a drain on your well-being. There is no maximum pain threshold you need to hit before you can leave a relationship.

One of the Gardeners, Samantha Saunders, 36, is a therapist, specializing in supporting high-achieving women, most of whom are in unfulfilling romantic relationships. The most common struggle her clients face, she told me, is recognizing the impact the relationship is having on them emotionally.

"To even be okay with this [toxicity] . . . you have to detach from yourself in some way," Saunders said. "When you have to keep numbing yourself, pushing your emotions down, or minimizing how you feel about it and keep pushing to the side, it's kind of like emotional constipation."

But the objective, Saunders told me, is to consider how the relationship *feels*. We tend to muddle over that part and go through all types of complex gymnastics to justify why we stay in spaces our mind and body are nudging us to leave. We want to believe the story we created at the beginning of the partnership, where we would learn and grow together and build something beautiful. After a bit of time, we're attached to this person and we want to believe the best-case scenario. Or, sometimes more plainly, we've invested considerable time and energy into this relationship. We don't want it to go to waste, the sunk cost fallacy be damned. All those tears must mean *something*.

But if you are crying every day, your heart sinks when they come home, you can't have a single conversation without it devolving into something stressful, your mind and body is registering all that upheaval. Your mental health will suffer.

We endure because we believe that if we just try a little harder—

read a different book, try a different podcast, say the hard things softer—the relationship will be different.

What complicates the matter is that in some cases, this is true! Relationships *can* be different if both parties are committed to doing the work involved in bringing a dying relationship back to life. I've seen (and experienced firsthand) many relationships pulled back from the brink, restored to a place where the nervous system (of both parties) can settle.

How can you tell if your relationship is salvageable? That's a hard call to make but ask yourself: *What percentage of your relationship was good before it turned? How long have you been in a downward spiral? Is trust, consideration, thoughtfulness present? If you were not in a relationship with them, would you be friends with them? How does your body react to their presence?* And perhaps the question that allows you to see your relationship most clearly—*would you want your daughter to be in a relationship like this?*

There's no checklist I can write that tells you when to push harder to make a relationship work or when to walk away because you've given your all. When it comes down to it, there's only three choices if you feel your relationship isn't working for you: *you can leave, you can stay in the same patterns*, or *you can change the dance.*

Leaving isn't always easy, I'll admit. You likely have a significant emotional investment in this relationship, even if it affects your mental health. However, your peace of mind is paramount in any relationship you find yourself in, especially the one that is in your home. If you feel like you want to leave but can't leave *today*, that's okay. Make your plan and work your plan.

Staying requires you to look clearly at your relationship *as it is* and decide for yourself that it is enough. If you think you may stay, determine your "Basic Standard of Care" within your relationship. Let's say emotional safety and financial security are paramount for you. Your partner checks off those two boxes, but at their core they are a homebody so you're always trying to get them to travel and have new experiences with you. Staying means you've decided the things they offer (perhaps stability and peace of mind) outweigh the things they don't (let's say, an adventurous spirit) and find other ways to get those needs met. You decide, actively, that what they offer is worth the sacrifice.

And finally, if you feel there's a solid foundation for growth and continued partnership, you can change the dance.

I'll be the first to admit that being expected to take the lead in fixing a relationship is exhausting. This burden usually falls on women, and I've always resented how the bulk of emotional labor is magically expected to be our responsibility.

However, in my marriage, I was tired of waking up with the weight of our troubles on my chest. I wasn't looking to leave but I was ready to end the cycle of discontent we found ourselves in, a dark gray cloud over most of our time together. When you're tired of having the same conversation over and over, you've got to find new ways of being.

What helped most was a reframe. I wasn't "fixing the relationship." I was putting myself in charge of my own experience within the relationship.

That meant I was required to show up differently for *myself*. Not for *their* benefit or *our* benefit but my own. I began to move in ways that prioritized my well-being—I went to the gym. I started reading more books (more than relationship advice titles). I started prioritizing laughter and watching comedy specials. I leaned on my girlfriends and found more joy in our meetups. I made myself a bit more physically unavailable at home to prioritize my peace. I journaled. I got back to doing things I loved just because I loved them. When it came to the relationship, I started to view us with an objective lens, as if I was responding *for* Tara, not *as* Tara. Almost like *Key & Peele's* Obama Anger Translator skit but in reverse.

If you've been in a downward spiral in your relationship for a while, chances are there are a few patterns you recognize. Someone criticizes, someone gets defensive. Someone seeks closeness, the other one turns away. Someone initiates conversations, the other one is conflict avoidant. Someone triggers the other person and the other person explodes.

Whatever your pattern, shifting *your* response changes the entire flow. If you typically get defensive, pause for a moment and acknowledge *something* that feels true about what your partner is saying. If you're the one who typically shuts down, offer a way for the conversation to continue, even if it can't happen right then.

Shifting your response is its own power. The only person in a relationship you can change is yourself. Taking charge of *your* behavior is truly the only path forward. Imagine the two of you are literally on the dance floor, doing the same moves you've been doing for years. Then one day, you grab your partner's hand and to their surprise, you go left when you usually go right. They might be slow to notice the change at first, but over time, they'll realize, *Hey, this is a new dance. We're in a new space.* Even if it doesn't shift the other person's behavior, it will give you greater peace of mind that the dance won't continue in the same way. You've done your part.

In time, these changes allow you to have the breathing room you need to make the bigger, long-lasting changes that keep your mental space clear.

No matter what you choose, find ways to get clarity on what is happening, whether that's by being open and vulnerable with a trusted friend or checking in with a mental health professional. You need a space where you can parse through what can stay and what must go.

Again I want to remind you: All the yoga and deep breathing and herbal teas won't matter if you don't feel peace in the place where you lay your head at night. You can't self-care your way out of an unhealthy relationship. It requires direct, intentional action to ensure your intimate spaces are as beneficial to you as possible. You deserve a love that nourishes you. *Period.*

QUESTIONS TO ASK YOURSELF

- What examples of healthy love (ones filled with care, affection, recognition, respect, commitment, trust, and honest communication) have I witnessed firsthand in my life?
- Do my partners' words align with their actions? Do my words align with my actions?
- What patterns am I seeing in this relationship? What role am I playing in these patterns?
- What does a healthy relationship look like for me? Does my current relationship qualify?
- What evidence do I have that my partner is just as invested as I am in improving this relationship?

TEND TO YOUR MENTAL AND EMOTIONAL WELLNESS

GROWING INTO WHO we were meant to be is a lifelong endeavor, beginning in childhood and following all the days of our lives. Tending to our mental and emotional wellness looks different in different seasons, but these items should remain constant throughout your life.

INSTITUTE YOUR OWN MENTAL HEALTH DAY POLICY

When do you get a break? How long can you go before your energy light starts blinking red? Whatever the frequency, make sure to catch yourself before the breakdown. Honor your time by giving it a name. My aunt calls her days off "pajama days." Whatever you do, give it a name. Sounds silly, but a name makes it real!

ALLOW ROOM FOR *EVERY* EMOTION

We mistakenly believe there are "good" emotions and "bad" emotions. We exalt certain emotions (joy, anticipation, courage, bravery) and hide others (sadness, anger, embarrassment, disappointment). But wisdom is knowing that each emotion is a crucial part of us.

INTERROGATE YOUR CAPACITY

We want to believe that our energy is limitless and we can do everything our mind tells us is possible. But being honest with our capacity and recognizing we are but one person, allows us to get real about what can stay on our plate and what must go.

SIT YOUR BURDENS DOWN

Where do you put your issues when they get heavy? Find a sacred space to be, whether that's therapy, a trusted friend or family member, a journal, a support group. Life is meant to be a team sport, sis. (Speaking of a team sport, perhaps it's time to analyze your inner circle. Flip to the social wellness chapter for a deeper dive.)

TILLING THE SOIL: MENTAL AND EMOTIONAL WELLNESS JOURNALING QUESTIONS

- What is my biggest current stressor?
- How do I release the biggest, messiest feelings I have?
- What activities do I need to unleash the unburdened side of me? What did I enjoy as a child?
- What do I need in my life to feel mentally and emotionally well?
- How do my closest relationships make me feel?
- What kind of reinforcements do I need in order to feel more comfortable with rest?

Honoring Our Creativity

CREATIVE WELLNESS

When I dance, I'm in this heightened place where all of those things that make me feel sad go away. I get to feel things on another plane. It's indescribable. It's almost as if I'm not here. I'm not present in this physical space, but I'm in another place where there's just joy. It's just purely joy. That's why when I'm not feeling well, I'm like, *I just wanna dance. Please. I'll get better. I'll get better if I could just dance and listen to some music.* It's heaven on earth.

—Talise Campbell, 48, dance educator and choreographer

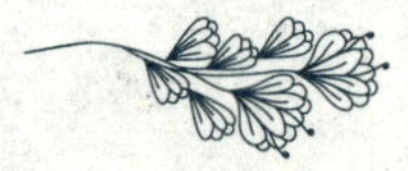

EXPLORING THE ROOTS

IN SUMMER 2020, a billboard in Los Angeles went up with an insightful tweet from writer Melissa Kimble, who proclaimed: "The world does not move without Black creativity."

Kimble had no idea she would see her words on a billboard.[1] Twitter executive Godis Rivera was working on a project to amplify Black voices, specifically those of the Black Lives Matter movement. At Rivera's request, Kimble sent over a couple tweets, thinking nothing of it.

A few months later, Oscar-winning director Matthew Cherry tagged her in a tweet that captured her billboard high above traffic on Beverly Boulevard in Los Angeles. Kimble was in awe. *Oh, and one more thing*, Rivera told her—there's also a billboard in Chicago, her hometown.

Kimble's words resonated for one major reason: Black creativity makes the world go round.

Our imagination and ingenuity are not just an American experience, but a major global export. It is the blueprint. Our minds shape and shift culture.

Everything you love about [*fill in the blank here*] is because of Black people. You can't listen to a movie trailer without hip-hop providing the soundtrack. The beauty industry would have nothing without Black girls to pull from. Our influence dominates in fashion, literature, food, speech, music—often without proper recognition.

Nikki Giovanni said it best: "If we can't drive, we will invent walks and the world will envy the dexterity of our feet. If we can't have ham, we will boil chitterlings; if we are given rotten peaches, we will make cobblers. If given scraps, we will make quilts; take away our drums and we will clap our hands. We prove the human spirit will prevail. We will take what we have to make what we need. We need confidence in our knowledge of who we are."[2]

Black creativity is a matter of lineage. Think of what we've been able to create *in spite of*. Being stripped of our language, our customs, our connections, we have had to start from scratch here in America. We retained what we could and built something new. We have always been able to look at something and imagine the missing piece. We have been blessed with the gift of possibility, of wonder, of curiosity. That creativity is a generational gift, a necessity.

Kimber Thomas, a native of Jackson, Mississippi, completed an oral history project on the art of "making do," her contribution to documenting the ingenuity of Black Southern women.[3] The women, all 70 years old and older, told stories of their mamas using forks as hot combs, old tobacco tins and strips of brown paper bags as hair rollers, mixing lard with lye to straighten their hair. This resilient creativity "served as the means by which these women defined freedom for themselves in the absence of sociopolitical freedom during the Jim Crow era." In another life, these women would be engineers, spending their days finding ways to problem solve for big paychecks. Instead, they used their know-how to shift the way they were seen as best they could.

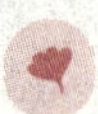

POET LUCILLE CLIFTON has been my creative muse through the writing of this book. The more I read her and the more videos I watched, the more I knew that she was my kind of people. We both grew up on the shores of Lake Erie, some forty years apart—her in Buffalo, New York, me farther south in Cleveland. That Rust Belt sensibility climbs into her work, the grit and resilience evident in poems like "homage to my hips" or "won't you celebrate with me?"

I read Clifton's "mulberry fields" just once before it imprinted directly on my heart. The poem, about grave markers of the enslaved that were removed in St. Mary's County, Maryland, to make way for the new State House, reflects the heart of the Black condition. We are often forgotten or bulldozed out of the way. Clifton, in all her creative prowess, would not let that happen on her watch. She used her pen to draft poems about life as an outspoken, Black, "luxury-sized woman," as she called herself.

But still, Clifton had a full life outside of writing. A mother of six, she wasn't convinced that her creative calling could be a full-time endeavor. But she found a way to do it all. Because she had to.

"When my first book of poetry came out, my kids were 7, 5, 4, 3, 2, and 1," Clifton said in an interview.[4] "I learned to write in my head. So by the time I get to paper, I'm a long way into the process."

Women like Clifton are a reminder that we *can and should* make room for creativity. That opportunity likely won't present itself all pretty, wrapped up with a bow. It's up to us to lean into the benefit of a creative outlet as we move through this life.

For most of our time here in America, to be focused on creating for the sake of creating—not laboring for someone else—was a luxury most of our foremothers could not afford.

Alice Walker mused in *In Search of Our Mothers' Gardens*:[5] "How was the creativity of the Black woman kept alive, year after year and century after century, when for most of the years Black people have been in America, it was a punishable crime for a Black person to read or write? And the freedom to paint, to sculpt, to expand the mind with action did not exist."

Walker's mother—Minnie Tallulah Grant—was an artist. Never mind that she was also a sharecropper with eight young children. Grant's creative medium of choice was the literal earth. Walker claimed her mother's growing prowess was "magic," producing gardens so lush and beautiful that strangers would stop to compliment the dahlias and delphiniums.

"Whatever rocky soil she landed on," Walker marveled, "she turned into a garden. . . . She is involved in work her soul must have."

That "soul work" is the heart of this chapter. What, among our busy lives, is our soul yearning to do? What can we create? I can imagine Grant humming to herself with her fingers knuckle deep in the dirt, just as I can imagine Clifton writing from a place of joy on her typewriter.

With increasing responsibilities, creative pursuits are often the first to get the axe from our schedule. How can we choose between a photography class and making sure our baby makes it to and from soccer practice?

But just because something is hard to fit into our lives doesn't mean we shouldn't try. We have to hold the door open for light to flow in. Creativity isn't just about making *things*. It's about making *us*. It is precisely those moments when we lose ourselves in the "flow" where we are reminded of what it means to be alive.

Our creativity shows up in our daily lives—the way we dress, how we choose our meals, how we decorate our living spaces, and such. All of it is self-expression, a way to say to the world "I'm here." You don't have to be an "artist" to be an artist.

At its core, creative wellness is reflecting the ways that *playfulness, freedom*, and *imagination* show up in your daily life. Our charge is to orchestrate more opportunities to live fully within their bounds.

Leaning into my creativity helps me mute my inner critic and turn the volume up on my inner cheerleader. It gives me a safe space to play in the muck, to remind myself *you don't have to take everything so seriously all the time.* Artistic expression is about finding the most honest part of yourself and pulling it outward. We aren't perfect people so our art won't be either. Through the process of creating, I can see the things I admire internally brought forth externally. Once you sink into it, you can remember exactly who you are. You can begin to shed expectations of perfection and instead live as you are.

I deserve to have a space to be imperfect and so do you.

Too many of the expectations of Black women are heavy, and frankly I'm sick of it. I want to experience a life where my smile—when and where and how often it appears—is the biggest indicator of my success. I want my days to be laced with joy.

I want that for you too.

WHO TAUGHT YOU ABOUT NURTURING YOUR CREATIVITY?

FOR MOST OF my life, my creative output was (surprise, surprise!) writing. I was a magazine fiend as a preteen. I loved *Suede* and *Honey* and *Vibe Vixen*, all published to guide me toward the woman I couldn't wait to be when I grew up: a sexy, confident boss. I'd pore over each issue, cover to cover, and imagine my name on the masthead. I would sit at the family computer and write magazine cover stories about myself, pretending I was a rapper signed to Bad Boy, mentored by Lil' Kim and best friends with Faith Evans (whew, that didn't age well *at all*).

The best way I knew how to express myself, an anxious, socially awkward little Black girl, was to sit at a computer and let my fingers dance over the keys. I would "play" Mavis Beacon Teaches Typing so I could type without looking down at the keyboard, because those few seconds were the difference between my fingers being able to keep up with the thoughts as they flowed out of my brain. After I won my first writing contest in elementary school, the award gave me the notion that *Hmm, this could be the thing for me.*

My parents nurtured the hell out of my writing, making sure I grew up in libraries and bookstores, and signing me up for youth journalism programs, even when I was reluctant to give up my Saturday mornings to participate.

I probably got the reading and writing bug from my father, who worked for a local Black newspaper during my toddler years. Every other creative endeavor I've pursued—crocheting, interior decorating—was directly linked to my mom.

Like many mothers of her era, my mother expressed much of her creativity through her children—the pink and white beads at the end of our braids, held in place by a scrunched piece of foil, perfectly matching our outfits. The pink and green wallpaper that she insisted I get for my room when she finally allowed me to redecorate as a teen. The pink frilly dresses she would select for Sunday church service. (Can you tell my mom is an AKA?) In every memory I have of my mother, she was busy, either with school or working multiple jobs. There wasn't a lot of room for her own creativity to manifest in ways that could be the center of her life, but it made itself known in ways we couldn't ignore. I learned that *creativity will grow in the cracks of our lives, if we let it.*

In my conversations with the Gardeners, creativity certainly wasn't a priority most could point to in their whole and busy lives. As I predicted, our discussions focused on work and family and taking the "safe and expected" route. But for some, their creative urges were going to take center stage, no matter what anyone else had to say about it.

Assia Pulliam-Richardson, 32, had a creative role model in her hairdresser mother. Growing up in Virginia, she dabbled in a little bit of everything, encouraged by her mom.

"When I was little, my granny would say, 'Oh, Assia is so destructive,' she told me. 'She's always breaking stuff or taking stuff apart.' And my mom would say, 'No, she's curious.' She would just let me explore, whether it was taking apart old electronics or bringing in plants and bugs from outside. I had the freedom to explore things. If it was interesting to me, go try it."

That freedom to follow her instincts paid off. After six years in the military, Pulliam-Richardson followed the tug to pursue her biggest dream: making it as an actress in Hollywood. Several films later, she credits her mom with giving her the confidence to make the leap.

"My mom was a free spirit, and she was all about doing what you want to do," she said. "The main thing I think I picked up from her was, if there's something that you wanna do, you do it. *You* are responsible for making whatever come to fruition."

But even if artistry and creativity are discouraged, it eventually finds a way to be known. Cleveland native Michelle Starling, 48, a visual artist and art therapist, told me her career goal was to "make art and help people." It took thirty years, but she got there.

"When I was younger, an undergrad, I wanted to major in art," Starling explained. "But my mother was like, 'No, if you're gonna be an artist, you can be an artist, but you need to have a steady profession.' So my undergrad [major] was in political science, pre-law."

After graduation, she found her way to the classroom, but she remained committed to art at heart. "I would always incorporate art into my lesson plans, my classroom. Artistically I was doing the proms, homecoming, every bulletin board, every wall in the place would have something of mine on there. And when that break would come, I would just unleash all of the creativity and go from there. It was freeing."

Her website is full of beautiful mosaic tile work. She picked up the medium after her uncle, a self-taught artist, died and his wife gave Starling all his materials and supplies. She dove into figuring out how to express herself through the multicolored tiles during winter and summer breaks.

Eventually, she couldn't restrict her creativity to school breaks. She enrolled in graduate school to become an art therapist, a field that is 99 percent white. Now, she spends her days working with Black women, encouraging them to put their armor down through group art therapy sessions.

"Every piece I do to honor my uncle, and I wish I would've started sooner. I wish I would've been able to make art with him. But everything happens for a reason. And for me, honoring him kind of pushed my work forward and made it more meaningful, more purposeful."

Creativity isn't something you have to seek—it is seeking you. Consider your younger self, whatever age you were before you learned of the external gaze, before you were worried about being judged for what you truly enjoyed. What did it feel like to create then?

Whether you learned art is something unpredictable or you were encouraged to be as creative as possible, there's time to lean into all your creative urges, I promise you.

WHO TAUGHT YOU ABOUT CREATIVE EXPRESSION?

- Do you remember your caregivers prioritizing creativity in any way?
- Was there space for you to play in your house, whether it was a bin for your toys or space in your room?
- Do you remember art classes in school? What projects come to mind? Did you or your parents keep the artwork you brought home?
- Were you a big reader as a child? Were other adults in your family?
- Do you daydream? What about?

RECLAIMING PLAYFULNESS

EVEN NOW AT 16, my son will enjoy a day at the park, swinging high on the swings, jumping off at the top with his teenage knees cushioning the fall. He'll spin other kids faster than he probably should on the merry-go-round and then jump on to enjoy the ride as well. At six feet tall (six three if you count his hair), he looks like a giant baby, full of joy and delight. He collects Transformers and loses himself for hours in Lego building sets. We often find ourselves roaming the toy aisles of some big-box store, where he will linger over what's new and encourage me to "feel the vibes."

When I found myself growing impatient in those aisles, I had to ask myself why. Just because I only came in here for deodorant and curtains doesn't mean I can't take a detour and browse the play aisles with my son. Now, nine times out of ten, I try to relax and enjoy the array of toys. My participation is a reminder to him that he doesn't have to age out of play.

Researcher Stuart Brown often resists giving a formal definition, but in *Play: How It Shapes the Brain, Opens the Imagination, and Invigorates the Soul,* he offers the following: "Play is the state of mind that one has when absorbed in an activity that provides enjoyment and a suspension of sense of time. And play is self-motivated, so you want to do it again."

Play is simple. It's less of an activity and more of a state of being. What gets you to zone out, lost in the fun of it? What do you gravitate toward, where no one has to force you to do it—you choose it willingly? *That* is play.

We need play in the same way we need to breathe, to laugh, to cry. Our play as adults might look a little different. Laughter is play. Joyful movement is play. Sex is play. Play is not easily defined, but you'll know when you have it.

We overlook all the ways play shapes us, both in childhood *and* adulthood. "Play creates new neural connections and tests them," Brown writes. "It creates an arena for social interaction and learning. It creates a low-risk format for finding and developing innate skills and talents."

Play is how children experience the world for the first time. They giggle, grab, wobble, explore. Babies aren't thinking ahead to what life is going to look like two weeks from now. They are strictly in the here and now, enjoying the sights and sounds in front of them.

Nothing has a distinct purpose other than discovering something new to get into.

But as we grow, we are expected to know what we are doing. We should have a clear view of the future and the responsibilities within. "Playing" is considered frivolous and a sign that you're not taking your responsibilities seriously enough.

That shift starts early. Most education policymakers know that play is crucial to child development—researchers would argue it is the number one way that children learn—and yet most schools phase out recess by middle school. Only nine states in the United States mandate daily recess.[6] Equipment at most playgrounds is built for the 12 and under set. Look at high school graduation requirements for your state—how many fine arts credits are recommended before students hit the "real" world. Not many, I can tell you that.

We learn early that playtime is over, even as the need for downtime and exploration remains constant.

"When we stop playing, we stop developing, and when that happens, the laws of entropy take over—things fall apart," Brown warns in *Play*. "When we stop playing, we start dying."

"I FEEL LIKE A KID AGAIN"

Years ago, I hosted a creativity workshop for Black women at my friend Da'Shika Street's creative art studio in downtown Akron, Ohio. It's a bright, spacious vibe, with a choose-your-own-adventure approach to art.

We chose to do splatter painting, which is just as it sounds. You sit your canvas on an easel, select paint colors, and fling paint at the canvas until you are satisfied with your piece.

The splatter area was sectioned off, and all attendees got protective gear. Street reassured the most skeptical of us that the paint was washable out of just about everything, a subtle nudge to let go of any worries or rigidity about what we were here to do. One by one we entered the splatter space, buoyed by our individual soundtrack selection.

As we began, there was hesitancy at first. "Oh, we're making a mess," we thought to ourselves. We had to sink into the moment, to remember that this wasn't a mess. This was *art*.

Splatter art ended up being the perfect activity to spark attendees' childlike creativity as they emerged with their paint-covered canvases, thrilled at the opportunity to not only let loose but explore what happened if they got close, if they stood farther away, if they flicked the bristles, if they loaded the brushes with paint versus a quick dip. What would happen if they smeared the paint with their fingers or used the brush handle to create lines?

Magic, that's what happened.

The goal was to offer a space to let go of any limitations we may have had on what our art "needed" to look like. As we finished, we looked around the table at our different pieces and admired what each attendee expressed on their canvas.

Street told me later that she opened her studio for women who needed a place where the responsibilities of life could melt away and be replaced by pure joy. An entrepreneur, wife, and mother to three, there are very few spaces in *her* life that aren't packed with obligations. She realized she needed a space like that for herself.

After a friend hassled her for months to join in the fun at the local skating rink and her husband unexpectedly purchased a pair of skates for her birthday, she finally obliged, not expecting anything more than a good time with a friend.

Instead, she found peace of mind—a place where pleasure was

the only thing that mattered. "I'm always trying to be in mom mode," she said with a sigh. "I'm trying to be a good example. I'm trying to be a leader. I'm trying to provide, I'm trying to teach life lessons. I'm trying to be a nurturer. I'm always trying to provide in all the ways my husband needs."

But when she skates, she said, none of that exists.

"It's a lesson on patience. It's a lesson on trusting myself. It's a lesson on what my capabilities are. It's a lesson that I can dance a little bit and groove and that's okay. If I were at home in my kitchen doing that, my kids would be laughing or making comments, but on the skating floor or at the rink, it's embraced. Other people high-five you. You find your people."

Listening to her talk, it forces me to be honest: It's really hard for me to get into the headspace to play. I'm often stiff and serious. Rigid in my ideas about what and when things are appropriate. I'm constantly aware of how I am being perceived in any given space, and my goal, at all times, is to be respected. For many years my round cheeks and short stature have led people to believe I'm a full decade younger than I really am, and coupled with my quest for respectability as a young mom, I have shifted the way I walk, talk, and dress. In short, sometimes I'm boring as hell. No playfulness to be found here.

Since I'm out of practice, I have to give myself "play models" to remind me to relax and not take everything so seriously. That's why I curate my social media experience to feature women like Nicole Goss, whose public performances as a Hula-Hoop flow artist take me back to elementary school, where all the girls spent the entire recess swirling their hips and showing off their skill. Goss's videos feature her hula-hooping all around Chicago, often in crowded spaces where onlookers stop and watch, most mesmerized by her fluidity and grace.

"I honestly don't mind when people watch from afar, especially children," she posted online.[7] "I have accepted that I am walking art and representation. Most have never seen someone use a Hula-Hoop the way we flow artists do and definitely have not seen a Fat Black Woman as myself twirling so freely. Also I love to see the smiles and looks of wonder. I get to bring joy by just doing me."

Artists like Goss serve as visual reminders that play is not optional.

Look at your footprint on a map. Over the last month, how many places did you visit that weren't work, school, or a store? How many detours in your normal routine did you take to infuse the day with some levity? Play opens our borders and allows us to reconnect with the woman under all the responsibility.

Don't you want to meet her?

What's your PLAY PERSONALITY?

Play researcher Stuart Brown names seven types of play personalities. Which resonates most with you?

- The Joker (practical jokes, pranks, silliness)
- The Kinesthete (movement as physical joy)
- The Explorer (new places, experiences, thoughts)
- The Competitor (joy driven by a desire to win)
- The Director (setting the scene, curating events)
- The Collector (gathering all their favorite items in one place)
- The Creator (using hands/heart/mind to create something)

A GOOD CACKLE

Black laughter is my favorite sound in the world. Something about it heals my soul.

I inherited my mother's laugh, which she inherited from her mother. My daughter not-so-affectionately describes it as a "witch's cackle." (Little does she know that she'll inherit that cackle from me in about a decade.) But I love our laugh because it comes from deep in the gut. When something is truly funny, I throw my head back and let the laughter erupt uncontrollably. I might even slap my knee for a little razzle-dazzle. When I stop, I'm amazed at how free it feels. I imagine my mother and grandmother having the same sensation of unbridled joy. I want to live in that moment forever.

Black laughter is my balm. You may have heard the saying that comedy equals tragedy plus time. We take pain and turn it into something we can look at without hurting our eyes.

One example: At our grandfather's memorial service, my sisters and I were sitting in our seats before the ceremony began, watching the slideshow of his life in photos, which I had painstakingly put together the week prior and set to his favorite gospel song, "Midnight Cry." It was designed to knock the tears right out of you without much effort. And the tears were indeed flowing, with us staring straight ahead at his urn and remembering the last time we saw him. He wasn't even sick. His death had been a complete shock to everyone in that room.

We were fortunate to have three grandfathers, courtesy of our grandmother's second marriage. Now all three were gone, each cremated and ashes placed among family members who wanted them.

As we sat and sniffled, my sister said solemnly, "Great. Now all we got left is Grandpa sand."

Grandpa sand? All three of us burst out laughing, tears running down our faces, the mood lightened enough that we got through the rest of the service with our hearts full. Black people know how to make a way outta no way, but we also know how to find the funny when shit looks bleak.

Writer Patia Braithwaite suggested that laughter is something of a weapon of mass resilience for Black folks.[8] "Laughter can make your shoulders shimmy. You might stomp, clap, or swat your neighbor's back. It's celebration and lamentation. It's release. It's also a battle cry against everyday anti-Blackness. It rejects the whispers to crouch down, fold into ourselves, or cover up. It refuses orders to be serious, to tighten our tongue. It resists pleas to be less vocal, less childlike—to be smaller, to be quiet. It connects us to each other without trying."

Laughter is a physiological process—when we laugh, our stomach contracts, our breathing changes. Our levels of endorphins (the feel-good hormones) increase and levels of cortisol (the stress hormone) decrease. Laughter will literally leave our bodies better than it found them.

That fact is not lost on Brandi Denise Boyd, an LA-based comedian who pursued comedy after leaning into her knack for making teachers and friends laugh. The evening before our call, she had been on the lineup with Mike Epps. As we spoke, she was driving to an audition she was convinced would go well. She tells me plainly: "I do comedy for Black women and if anybody else gets on board, great, but literally it's for us."

I gotta know, I asked her. *How does it feel to come offstage after you know you killed your set?*

"It's a sense of euphoria," she explained. "It's obviously a serotonin boost. Sometimes it's almost like an out-of-body experience. I get addicted to the confidence that I exude onstage. Because sometimes I have shows and I might not be the crowd's favorite, but I feel so good about myself."

As we talked, I wondered if she faced any resistance from her family on pursuing comedy full-time. She laughed at the thought.

"I could have told my mom I was gonna ride dirt bikes. She would've been like, *Yes, you are*. She just had this thing of like, try everything. Figure out what you want to do. This is what led me ultimately to comedy. Because even in college, I was doing spoken word, I was going onstage, I was doing background singing. I went and recorded some tracks in the studio. I was doing talent shows, and I think that was because my mother and my father were so supportive as a child and allowed me to do whatever I wanted to try."

Other folks, mostly college friends, didn't quite understand her experimentation. The message was clear—pick a lane and stick to it. Even though we're chatting over the phone, I can practically hear Brandi shrug.

"In college, my friends were like, *You all over the place, you always doing everything*. I did everything that crossed my mind that I wanted to do. If you're not hurting nobody, then you're okay. You can do whatever you want to do. It's your life."

I let Brandi hop off the phone to hopefully kill it at her audition, and her last words stayed on my mind. *It's your life*. I needed to hear that and maybe you did too.

❦

FINDING FREEDOM

POTTERY HAS BEEN my outlet for creative expression, but it didn't start that way. I signed myself up for a beginners' pottery class and sat down at my wheel ready to make a whole heap of bowls and mugs. I was convinced that I would be able to walk away with a good number of items to put on display at my home.

Toward the tail end of the first class, our instructor walked through the space, quietly observing me and my classmates hunched over the pottery wheels, struggling to keep our clay upright and centered. She stopped by my wheel and watched me silently for a few minutes before offering an observation.

"You're a bit of a perfectionist, aren't you?"

My cheeks got hot as she called me out. I got lost in the zone trying to ensure that my very first pot was perfect coming off that wheel.

Then she said the thing I wished she hadn't—she singled me out to give me praise in front of the rest of the class. *How did she know I had a praise kink?* I wondered. They turned their attention to my wheel and saw my first bowl hit all the marks she mentioned during her demo. I had managed to center the clay correctly so the sides and bottom were an even thickness, and it was sturdy enough to come off the wheel without an issue.

It was indeed perfect but it was one-third the size of everyone else's. Once it dried, it would shrink even more. After it was glazed and fired, it would shrink again in the kiln and wouldn't be good for anything other than a couple tablespoons of dip or a few pieces of jewelry.

I was still proud of the bowl, but I realized in that moment that

I was holding myself to an impossible standard, in a setting where perfectionism was as far from the goal as you could get. We were literally playing in mud and yet I still wanted to get an A plus in mud bowl making. (Somebody pray for me.)

Who was I failing if I didn't get it right on the first try? What would have been the consequence if I, like some of my other classmates, just got a feel for the clay that first session and took time getting to know how it reacted to certain pressures of our hands and speeds of the wheel?

I did just that during the second lesson and found the practice much more liberating than trying to "win" at pottery. I didn't have to be the best at something to enjoy it.

That art class was a victory in my lifelong battle with perfectionism, the practice of being exceptional at finding fault. It's not always a yearning to be perfect but always being conscious of how you and others around you are falling short.

To be fair to myself, this perfectionism didn't come from nowhere. Instead, it's been carefully honed over the years—as the eldest daughter trying to serve as a "good influence" for my younger sisters; as a journalist trained to craft stories with pinpoint accuracy and zero typos; as a mother raising two Black children. Most of my life is a tightrope, trying to avoid missteps for the sake of survival.

It's a delicate dance and I'm tired of the choreography.

LEANING INTO VULNERABILITY

One day I was scrolling Instagram and saw my friend Andrea Johnson—who I primarily know as a fierce community activist and leader of social change workshops—announcing her new project. Her debut single, "Shine," was now available to stream on all platforms.

Wait, hold on. I scrambled over to Spotify to listen. My ears were intrigued from the first verse: *Please tell me why / You fantasize and dream but you don't try / It's almost like / Your doubts are in the driver's seat of life.* Her sweet, slightly husky voice rides the catchy dance beat that builds and builds into an anthem of self-love and a rejection of impostor syndrome.

Coming from a musical family, Johnson, 30, grew up with song lyrics churning through her body, depending on her nightly music to lull her to sleep. She couldn't remember a time when music wasn't playing in her ears and heart.

But that love of music meant she was well-versed in Whitney's powerhouse vocals, Mariah's whistle register, Beyoncé's husky Southern runs. Leaning into her gift meant she would have to listen to her own voice—the true definition of an artist.

"My voice is mine for a reason," she told me. "I'm not supposed to sound like everybody else. 'Cause I'm not everybody else. I have this desire to sing and to share my voice and my art and my thoughts and my feelings for a reason. That desire is a good thing. I don't have to fit."

Singing is so incredibly intimate, I told her. *It takes a lot of courage to release your voice into the world, doesn't it?*

"Part of my gift to this world is my vulnerability and sharing my experience," she said. "On a basic level, when we share our stories, other people get to see their own stories in that and affirm their own stories or feel a story that they haven't yet felt, or they had been avoiding in themselves or just hadn't had the space for. Our capacity to feel especially our pain sits at the root of so many of our world problems—systemic, societal, economic. I feel like so much of it comes down to like our capacity to be with our pain with ourselves and each other and tend to that pain."

When we caught up with each other, she had just performed the longest solo show of her career at Chicago's Uncommon Ground, a venue for indie artists to perform and build their audience. Admittedly nervous, she knew there was plenty of love in the audience to carry her through her set. "When I get up in front of people, for the most part, they're like, *I wish I could do that*," she said. "Opening myself up to receiving that love and that care that everybody in that room just wanted to be with me as I shared my art with them . . . it was so beautiful. I cried all the way home."

That vulnerability to stand onstage, plant her feet, and *sing* reminded Johnson that she was doing exactly what she was meant to do.

Talking with Johnson made me recall a 1968 interview with singer Nina Simone, in which an off-camera interviewer asks her to reflect on the definition of freedom.[9] "What's 'free' to me? Same thing it is to you—you tell me," she jostles with the interviewer for a moment. A few moments later, she changes course, as if the answer was being downloaded in real time. She almost leaps out of the frame to share.

"I'll tell you what freedom is to me—no fear," the icon says, the intensity of her statement hanging in the air for a beat. Her voice softens. "I mean really, no fear. If I could have that half of my life . . . no fear." The thought is so powerful she has to steady herself with her hand. "Lots of children have no fear, that's the only way I can describe it. That's not all of it, but it is really something to feel no fear."

Fear sets in when we are focused on the consequences of being seen, even as being seen is the thing we want most in this world. What a predicament for our gentle souls.

Fear in our creative endeavors may sound like: *Who am I to do this? I don't have time to devote to this. I'm not really a creative person.*

The only way to push past the fear is to know it intimately. "Hello Fear," you may say. "What are you here to tell me?"

Your Fear may look smaller when you look directly at it. Or it may loom over you, seemingly impossible to shrink to a manageable size. In either case, your Fear has a message: *I'm afraid I am not good enough. I'm afraid to reveal who I really am. I'm afraid of standing in the light.*

Pushing past Fear means you look at it, nod your head to acknowledge its presence, and move forward anyway. Over time, Fear will learn that everything it believes—the self-doubt, the unworthiness—is a lie. Or at the very least, that Fear don't stop the show.

No fear, Simone tells us. Can you imagine?

CULTIVATING IMAGINATION

I'VE KEPT A copy of Natasha Marin's *Black Imagination* within arm's reach since it was published. The book was born after her viral 2016 *Reparations* project, in which people of color could identify material and immaterial needs that privileged white people could then fulfill.

However, perhaps predictably, she spent the next two years inundated with racist threats. *Black Imagination* was her attempt at personal reparations, to give back to her life some form of power after the onslaught of negativity hurled her way. The book gathered Black people of all ages, genders, abilities, sexualities and presented them with three prompts: *What is your origin story? How do you heal yourself? Imagine a world where you are loved, safe, and valued.*

I want to imagine a world where Black women are universally loved, safe, and valued. I want that world to exist already. We're four hundred years overdue.

For many in her book, that last prompt was unexpectedly difficult to answer. "Even when I attempted to imagine my made-up world, the magic was fleeting and that in itself makes me want to weep," contributor Adrienne La Faye offered. "I thought it would be fun, until I couldn't see my possibilities even in my imaginary mind."

For me, a world where I am loved, safe, and valued means I can move through the world with no armor. I would feel loved if my needs and desires were to matter to everyone who loved me. I would feel loved if I was greeted with things I needed before I knew I needed them. I would feel safe if, when I step outside my door, I am greeted with smiles. People ask me if I need help with anything. Friends, neighbors, relatives all exist peacefully within my ecosystem and we simultaneously give and take as we need. I would feel safe if my children were safe. I would feel valued if my effort to make this world better was seen for what it is.

What would make you feel safe, loved, and valued? This thought exercise stretches our imagination. Training your imagination is like any other muscle—you use it or you lose it. Some of us are horribly out of shape imaginatively. We can't see past today to envision tomorrow. Our daydreams are less daydreams and more movement through a checklist.

My imagination fuels all that's good in my life. My children? I saw them first, even as I was ambivalent about motherhood. My career? I built this from scratch, with an inkling that one day I would be sitting here, enjoying the fruits of my labor. My marriage? I saw it unfold in my mind, planning our ten-year anniversary party before the end of the first year of matrimony. My friends? I cultivated them, one by one, because I knew they were solid people to keep in my orbit.

What I'm asking you to do is to rev up your imagination. I'm asking you to consider a world in which things are different from the one you currently occupy. It's a tall order some days, when our hope is low and we are downright exhausted from the actual reality we experience. But imagination is the first step. We have to envision what we want to see before we can know what steps to take to get there.

In *Imagination: A Manifesto*, professor Ruha Benjamin argues that imagination is a tool of liberation.[10] "It should be clear by now that our collective imagination has been arrested and confined, making it difficult to think beyond the racist, classist, sexist, ableist status quo," Benjamin wrote. "Those of us who refuse to accept oppressive ideologies show us what is possible when we unleash our imagination. We can rob unjust systems of their power and make a way outta no way—imagining different possibilities for how to connect and care for one another as we also remake the world."

Everything, she reminds us, is made up. One day, humans decided that *this* should exist and now it does. Our imagination is powerful beyond measure.

If we give ourselves an opportunity to imagine, we can paint with colors we didn't know existed.

MOTHERHOOD DON'T STOP NO SHOW

Tanikia Carpenter, 40, had only ever envisioned a creative career. As a young girl growing up in Chicago, she wanted to be Rudy from *The Cosby Show*. A writer and voracious reader, her goals shifted only slightly as she grew: She went from solely being an actress to expanding into being a playwright.

After she got married and was blessed in her thirties with her daughter, India, she tried to keep pushing and not miss a beat. When her daughter was 3 months old, Carpenter was cast in the play *Comfort Stew* at Chicago's ETA Theater. Determined not to let motherhood derail her like it had so many others, Carpenter felt she was up for the task. "I was in the green room pumping, literally giving my milk to the stage manager. Like, can you put this in the refrigerator please?"

I'm amazed that you were able to remember your lines, I joke with her. My brain fog was so bad when I was in the early postpartum period. It would have turned into improv on that stage.

"I felt like I had something to prove because you hear people say, M*otherhood changes you, da da da*. I look back like, W*hat were you doing?*" Carpenter laughed. "Why were you gone from Tuesday to Friday, rehearsing from six to nine? What were you doing? Crazy."

As we spoke, Carpenter was preparing a new play, *Emmett's Photo*, about *Ebony* editor-in-chief John H. Johnson's decision to publish Emmett Till's picture after his brutal murder in Mississippi. Like most Black folks in Chicago, she has roots in the South, and she's been eager to explore Black history by putting it onstage, the one place that "always feels like home."

Carpenter learned, like many artists before her determined to juggle motherhood and creative expression, that her path is going to require a particular type of imagination to help her dreams come to fruition. That's not necessarily a bad thing. "I grew up reading Terry McMillan and watching her interviews. And I remember she said she had to go out to the mountains to write, and I just like held on to that like, man, I need to go to the mountains, or like Malibu to write." Her husband, a musician, gave her some words of wisdom: *You may be able to go write on a mountain one day, but right now it's about getting it in where it fits in*.

It was like a light bulb went on for Carpenter.

"I had been waiting for this perfect opportunity to get away from her so I can write and get away from the responsibilities of the house. And I gotta push through it right now. I have to find a way to incorporate my life now with her. Maybe I'll get up earlier or I'll structure this time, but I cannot *not* do it because this is what I'm called to do."

Our conversation shifts to Pauletta Washington, who most folks know as Denzel Washington's wife, without giving her recognition as a working actress in her own right. Carpenter had met the actress at the closing of *The Piano Lesson* on Broadway, where her son John David Washington was in a lead role. When Carpenter approached her and asked for a photo, Pauletta seemed surprised.

Most folks mob Denzel, Carpenter said, but she was determined to give the actress her flowers for both her acting prowess and her immense professional sacrifice. "I don't know if she did it gracefully, but she made the decision to say to Denzel, you go out there and get it and I'll raise the kids. And now she's getting back into acting and she seems happy to me. She doesn't seem like *I could have had the Oscars* but it was important for her to stay home and raise her children."

Carpenter answers my question before I can ask it. "Me? No, I'll be bitter," she said with a laugh. "I will be sending divorce papers probably, like that is not what I can handle. Women have to figure out what is best for you and your household and what can you live with if you cannot live without pursuing this dream. Because I work, but I'm also very actively pursuing writing and acting on the side. I believe this is gonna take over."

For now, Carpenter is enjoying imagining a future where anything is possible, where her husband and daughter will be front row at whatever production she's involved in. Chasing the dream might take a little longer but that's okay. The dream remains the dream, all the same.

IMAGINATION IN REAL LIFE

Taking in the work of visual artist a'driane nieves requires you to steady your feet.

My favorite of hers is a piece titled *Reimagining the Possibility of Home Being a Safe Place Within My Own Body.*[11] I'm one of those people who can never quite express how artwork makes them feel, but the best way I can describe this piece is to say she put *this is what it feels like to heal* on canvas. It vibrantly captures the sensation of shedding the old and embracing the new.

We first crossed paths in the online postpartum space, connecting over our shared love of Beyoncé and *The Mindy Project*. As I've known her I've been able to watch her grow her name as a full-time artist and outspoken activist.

A mom of three, nieves, 42, began her work nearly twenty years ago to find her way through postpartum depression. She picked up a brush and let the emotions spill onto the canvas. Nieves likens the work to a relationship where she can let her hair down and be fully, authentically herself.

"I can pour all of who I am into my art, into my paintings, and it can take it, and it doesn't expect or demand anything back in exchange for doing so," she shared.

She began working at a table in the dining room, keeping her supplies nice and tidy. Once they moved to a new house, she claimed a spare bedroom as her studio. As her work began to outpace the space and garner more attention, she moved from the bedroom to the garage.

The extra square footage gave her permission to go large in her work. She graduated from small canvases at the local craft store, to purchasing large rolls of canvas that she tacked up on her garage wall, fully covering the space.

Occasionally nieves shares her process on Instagram. As a fellow fun-size woman, I notice how she stretches and uses her entire body to reach the ends of her canvas. She moves in time with the music in her ears, sometimes a bit of Prince, sometimes Santigold. Watching her create is mesmerizing.

"It's a very full-body immersive physical experience," she said. "I'm stretching my arms as high as they can go. I am bending and contorting my body in different ways. I'm lunging. All of those things have really just helped me understand what it means to take up space. Especially when you have all of these intersecting identities. I'm a woman. I'm Black. I'm neurodivergent. I'm a mother. I'm an abuse survivor."

The canvas can hold all of her, a safe space for anything she needs to express.

My girl is solidly international—her work has been exhibited in Los Angeles, Tokyo, London. But her next challenge is an exhibition in France, where curators have tasked her with thinking BIG—creating a piece that is 32 feet high by 32 feet wide. That's roughly three stories tall by the length of a city bus. The prospect is daunting, nieves admits, but she's stretching to meet the moment.

"I'm working at a scale that is completely foreign to me. It's probably the most challenging project that I've had to date. It's my first museum show, and it's a lot. It's terrifying."

I do my best in the moment to assure nieves she has what it takes. She looks as if she believes me.

The key to imagination is to remember that we don't have to start from scratch. Every artist, every singer, every writer has built on what has come before them. In nieves's case, she knows creating her mural at that size is possible. She's taking cues from Black abstractionists like Julie Mehretu and Mark Bradford, whose international showings require precision and forethought as they prepare to create for enormous rooms they've never seen before.

"I'm very curious to see how I respond to that and how I'm able to accomplish it physically, let alone emotionally and mentally," nieves said. "But I am excited to see how I push myself to take up that much space."

Her imagination is the thing to get her there.

This chapter exists to remind you that you are more than work. You are more than simply surviving and keeping the lights on, even if that's your present reality. To change anything, we have to first imagine how it looks.

Leaning into our creative gifts forces us to contend with all our internal struggles. I don't know if that's enticing or frightening to you but I do know that in the future, it is going to be art that saves us and keeps us tethered to each other. That's the safe space, where all the goodness resides. Our full humanity exists there, without apology. Let's sink into it.

TEND TO YOUR CREATIVE WELLNESS

SOME OF US find it in song, others express it through dance, others paint and sew and create beautiful accessories. Whatever it is, our creative energy sustains us when life feels hard. Here's a few tips for cultivating creativity even in the midst of a full life:

FIND YOUR MUSE

Find somebody whose creativity sparks your own. For me, that's Natalyn Bradshaw, a multidisciplinary artist whose words always soothe when I read them. Follow them online or show up (in person!) to one of their events. Proximity to creativity begets creativity, always.

RELEASE JUDGMENT

We often think our art is not really "art." It's not good enough. We're not "doing it right." But art is one space where there is no right way. It's only your way. And don't we all need more of that? Give yourself permission to explore without judgment. Create without considering what anyone else thinks of what you made.

DABBLE

We don't have to commit to art the same way we commit to our families, our jobs, our responsibilities. There's no shame in being a dabbler. We can paint something one week, take a belly dancing class the next, and try candle making the following week. Who cares! Do what calls to you. Don't limit yourself!

BRING BACK RECESS

What can you do for thirty minutes during the day that feels fun? The only rule: It's got to be something that you enjoy and look forward to. Recess may look like sketching people as you sit at a park, or getting down and dirty with some finger paint. Whatever it is, give yourself the gift of play, of losing track of time immersed in something you love.

DAYDREAM

Lean back on a firm surface and let it hold you while you allow your mind to wander and daydream. My favorite prompt: *A conversation with myself ten years in the future. What is she doing? What does she want me to know? What does her life look like?* I allow myself to imagine all sorts of goodness. Practice calling forth your own goodness through the art of daydreaming.

TILLING THE SOIL: CREATIVE WELLNESS JOURNALING QUESTIONS

- Who is the most creative person you know? What do you admire most about them?
- Do you have a previous hobby that you abandoned somewhere in your earlier life? How could you make your way back to it?
- How do you choose your outward self-expression (jewelry, shoes, clothes, makeup, hairstyles/color)? What aspect of your aesthetic speaks most closely to who you are?
- Where is playfulness lacking in your life?
- What are your big, outrageous goals for the next ten years?

8

In Full Bloom

I don't want us to center the outcomes that are best for everybody else as we center our self-care. Those are by-products. When Black women center themselves and move from that space, we create more, we are more full, we're whole, we're coming to situations at 100 percent, not 20 percent. We've been running on E, 10 percent, 5 percent. Imagine us at a hundred. We are enough of a motivation to do it for ourselves, knowing that other people will benefit. I feel really clear about that. Black women being free sets everyone else free. And me being free for myself is enough. I want to make sure I say that.

—Stephanie Ghoston Paul, 33, coach and speaker

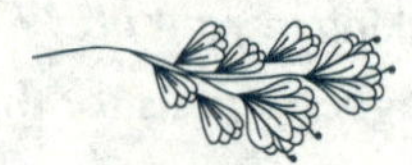

PICTURE YOURSELF IN the line of your ancestors.

Ahead are all the women who came before you. Your mother, her mother, her mother's mother. Stretching out beyond the horizon, each woman carrying the weight of her life as best she could, carving out moments for replenishment in a world that was determined to deny her.

Now turn around and picture yourself at the head of your line of descendants. All those who came after you, whether from your bloodline or from your connections with those you love. They're looking to you, wondering how you managed to navigate your life's biggest moments. Your life is their inspiration.

That's incredible power within your grasp. You're able to influence generations of women with how you move through the world. Whether you say "no" when you really mean "no." Whether you take the mental health day. Whether you deliberately remove yourself from relationships that are draining. Whether you release your emotions or keep them bottled up.

Let that power inspire and encourage you to step more boldly into who you desire and deserve to be. It's not meant to be placed on your shoulders lightly. This whole book serves to remind you that your life matters to more people than just yourself.

START HERE

AFTER ALL THE stories and discussion placed before you in this book, I'm sure you're wondering: *But where do I start?*

The simple answer: I'm willing to bet you already know.

Consider what it means to bloom as plants do: to emerge from a dark, cramped space but with the knowledge that you have all the material you need to perform as you were intended to.

Over the last decade I've spent most of my time planning and executing events around the country, all with the goal of bringing Black women together in a room to learn *from each other*, to heal *with each other*. I try to get out of the way and let the conversation unfold in a manner that gets them where they need to be.

Often, we don't need to be led. We don't need someone to stand at the front of the room and tell us how to live, how to maintain, how to thrive. We already know. The problem is that life is so demanding that we typically don't have the mental space or the emotional bandwidth to consider the task. We can figure it out once we create the space. That's what this chapter is about—making room.

I offer you this: Close your eyes and take a few calming breaths. Really take a minute to ground yourself. Now answer the following question:

In one year, what about your life would you like to be completely different and what would you hope is exactly the same?

It's easier to answer if you're able to be honest with yourself. What do you spend your time worried about? What do you thoroughly enjoy? What part of your life do you wish you could bottle up to enjoy whenever you want? Where are you yearning for your life to expand?

Take a moment to sketch your ideal life through the six pillars of wellness on page 263:

Social (What do you envision as your ideal relational life?)	Creative (How do you envision the best way for you to tap into your creative forms of self-expression?)
Physical (What do you see as the best way to tend to your physical body, providing it nourishment and pleasure?)	**Professional** (How do you envision the way you will support yourself financially?)
Spiritual (How will you connect to a higher power and tap into your purpose?)	**Mental/Emotional** (What rituals or routines will ensure you stay mentally or emotionally well?)

Another way to approach this: Flip back to the quiz from the first chapter. If you didn't complete it, take ten minutes to review it now.

I told you previously that there's no *true* scoring, but I want you to look at the quiz and tell me what your goals are for each statement. Do you want to feel connected to your purpose? Your sense of style? Get great sleep? Have friends you can count on for anything? Let that be your guide as you answer your "Fast-Forward One Year" question.

As I was growing up, everyone would always ask about your five- or ten-year plan. I always found that question daunting and even more so now as I have two decades of adulthood behind me. This is why the "Fast-Forward" question only takes us 365 days into the future. A year is just long enough to make most changes you desire, without having to step on the gas relentlessly. It also provides enough urgency without losing sight of the goal.

Once you've discovered the answer, leave it on the paper and sleep on it. Return to it in the morning after you've had a good night's rest. The next step is to call in reinforcements. A shift will require more than just your own energy. It will take a team. If you don't have a team, add "community building" to your answer. But I bet if you slow down, get brave and vulnerable, you can find the team you need, closer than you think.

TEND TO YOUR GARDEN (BATTLING BURNOUT)

I'M WILLING TO bet that the majority of you reading this book have experienced or are currently experiencing some level of burnout. We're living through unprecedented times. Every single day the headlines remind me that life is fleeting and unpredictable. Which is why, again, the care and keeping of our minds, bodies, and souls must be priority number one because this world will take us out of here if we let it.

I'm not going down without a fight.

While burnout is heavy and can feel like walking through mud, it can also be a gift. Burnout is our mind and body's check engine light, guiding us to slow down and pay attention to the pace and fullness of our lives. The longer we resist those signals, the deeper the hole we have to dig ourselves out of.

My check engine light had been staring me in the face for a smooth year after my layoff. I had thrust myself into freelancing while parenting full-time and balancing the remainder of graduate school. After working on all cylinders for more than two years, I was starting to feel it. It seemed like most of my friends were drowning at the same pace so I couldn't look to them as a life preserver. My marriage was going through growing pains, and I was at a complete loss as to how to get it back on track. I spent too many days getting to five in the afternoon completely exhausted, yet unsure of what I had actually accomplished. I had reached a boiling point in everything. Something had to give or I wasn't going to make it out.

I felt aimless, depleted, and overwhelmed.

Recovering from burnout is about creating room. It's about streamlining and removing responsibilities from our plate, yes, but it's also about inviting more juicy goodness in. It's releasing and welcoming at the same time.

This entire book is a perfect companion for burnout recovery, taking you bit by bit through each area of your life so you can analyze how to get more peace and calm across the board.

CREATE IMMEDIATE ROOM

In this first step, something has to give. Often when I coach women through bouts of burnout, there's a resistance. How could things possibly change? Everything that stresses us now will always stress us, it seems. Ask yourself: *In a perfect world, what would give me the most relief? What is possible for me?*

PROTECT YOUR ENERGY

Now more than ever it's critical to talk about how to practice intentional energy management. My method for the past few years is the "If/Then" strategy, which is all about keeping that energy balance in check. Every time you engage in something that you know is going to be draining, it's up to you to figure out a way to replenish yourself. In practice, it looks like this:

IF I have a three-hour Zoom call, THEN I will order takeout or eat leftovers so I don't have to wear myself out in the kitchen.
IF I deep clean the kitchen, THEN I will kick my feet up the rest of the day.
IF I stay up late to finish this project, THEN I will sleep in on Saturday.

If/Then is about sitting with your capacity and understanding that what goes out must come back. Otherwise, you're running yourself into the ground *on purpose*. Self-neglect ends here.

CREATE BLANK SPACE

You must have time in your day when you are doing nothing. I don't mean when you are transitioning from one thing to another. That's still *something*. I want you to have portions of the week where you don't have a single person calling you, depending on you, requiring you to show up somewhere and expend energy on their behalf. If you don't have this, the clutter of your mind will continue to clank around in your brain, looking for an exit. The silence and space you give yourself is the exit.

ADD JOY AND REPEAT

What lights up your world? Is it laughter with a friend? Time on the beach? Painting? Singing? What does your life need to feel lighter? What puts a smile on your face without you thinking about it? To paraphrase Alex Haley, find the joy and prioritize it.

HOLD THE SPACE

After a few months of creating room and adding more joy to your life, you may begin to feel better. You may cry less or have more energy. You may begin to see the world in color again. At this point, you may feel like things are looking up. Your boundaries and space-holding might get a little lax. But I'm here to remind you to *hold tight.* A full recovery from burnout could take anywhere from six months to three years, depending on the severity. Give yourself time to heal.

If you're like many of the women I've been in community with over the past decade, you might have read this entire book and felt intimidated, instead of invigorated, by the prospect of implementing so many changes into your life.

Caring for yourself is a full-time endeavor, yes. It requires energy and intention. Imagination and determination. It can be a simple thing to put yourself on autopilot, gritting your teeth as you get through the days. Some prefer it even.

But I think back to what life felt like when I didn't have my hands on the wheel. Perpetually tired and dragging through the days.

Every day I have to make a choice between my old way of living (getting by) and my new desire of living a full, meaningful life where I thrive.

I had to change how I viewed myself—from a woman whose worth was in how she served others to a woman who didn't have to "prove" anything to anyone. That's hard.

So believe me, I hear you. This journey requires a complete mindset shift so that *eventually* . . . it gets easier. Eventually, you will begin to shed old habits and replace them with new rituals that keep you focused, balanced, and joyful.

It's hard . . . until it ain't. Let's get free together.

GROW IN COMMUNITY (BEING A WOMAN WHO RECEIVES)

NEEDING SOMEONE TO watch your kids or help you around the house or support you as you grow your career—these aren't signs of weakness. Needing someone to walk through life with you—whether it's a partner, a nanny, an employee, a good friend—is not a flaw. It's not something you should apologize for. As my friend Alex once told me, "It's perfectly okay to try to make life easier for yourself." And sometimes, making life easier for yourself means calling in reinforcements so you don't have to carry your stress alone.

Some quick homework: Take a moment to make an informal list of all the people who you admire. This could be people who you know in real life or celebrities. Ask yourself, *Do they do everything solo or do they have help?*

I'm guessing you already know that answer. So what makes you any different?

If you still have trouble asking for help, let's solve this once and for all.

"I've been let down before."

None of us have support systems that will always hit the mark, no matter how much we might wish otherwise. But sometimes that disappointment helps us refine our approach. Did we ask the wrong person? The right person but at the wrong time? Were we clear in our ask?

"I actually don't know what I need."

This is more common than you think! If you're struggling to identify your needs, journal a bit. Imagine your load being lighter and your days a little brighter. What needs to happen in order to feel like that?

"I don't want to be a burden."

This has to do more with our own self-image and how we decide who is worthy of care. Take some time to sit with this imagery of "being a burden." What does that look like? How often can you ask for help before it becomes "burdensome" to those you love? Do you think you've even come close to hitting that imaginary mark?

LET'S STAY ON that "burden" conversation for a minute: We all know somebody who is an energy vampire. Every time you talk to them, they are asking for a favor or talking your ear off about their lives without asking how you're doing or if it's a good time. With them they take too much. The relationship feels one-sided. And because we know that person, we don't want to *be* that person. You don't want another person to look at you and think, "She's too much."

But here's the good news. You don't have to worry about being a burden if you recognize that other people have a responsibility for their own boundaries and capacity.

That energy vampire? Perhaps they could reflect on their own behavior and look at the ways they don't move in reciprocity. But you don't have to consent to them draining you. Ultimately, it's your responsibility to draw those boundaries.

It can be helpful to sit down and think about why you are hung up on asking for help (which will allow you to tackle that issue so you can request assistance with ease), but another tactic is to simply get in the habit of asking for help.

Skip all the whys and hows and "I'm uncomfortable" and just . . . do it. We often find we are more comfortable paying for help (if we need it). And while money can solve a lot of our problems, a limited budget shouldn't mean we suffer in silence and overwhelm. Depositing care into your community means there will be times when you give and there will be times when you receive. Being in community brings balance.

One day one of my best friends was in a bind and didn't have anyone to watch her 2-year-old daughter during an important lunchtime event at her art studio. She sent me a quick text asking if I could step in. I was delighted.

I showed up to her studio a few minutes before the guests were scheduled to arrive. She was a little frazzled, as to be expected, but she was prepared and ready to kill it. "Thank you for helping," she said as she rummaged in her purse for her debit card. She suggested that I take her daughter to the pizza shop next door for a couple slices. As we headed out the door, it hit me that I had everything that was important to her at that moment: her daughter and access to all her money. *Oh, we friends for real, for real,* I thought to myself with a chuckle.

I took her daughter to get some food and we walked around the neighborhood for an hour, until the little one got tired and I carried her back to her mom. It was truly invigorating. What a gift she gave me, to show up and embody love in action. I'm reminded of that moment every time I hesitate to ask a friend for support. When community is true, support is joyous. My bestie Amber is big on reminding me that supporting me and showing up for me is easy. "What an honor," she tells me regularly. It's enough to make my shoulders relax and any asks I have come easier.

We heal in community. We grow in proximity to others.

When we're focusing on getting through the days and we're buckling under the weight of everything on our plate, often we are too isolated and not moving as someone in community.

A lot of us are doing work solo that is meant to happen within our networks. We're not meant to be parenting children without backup. We are not meant to climb the career ladder without a mentor. We're not designed to carry the weight of our whole lives by ourselves, leading to mental and emotional strain. We're walking around here wondering why life feels so damn hard. It's not you, sis! It's the empty slots in your life where your help is supposed to be.

Let's make it plain: Any self-care or wellness routines that rely solely on your singular efforts will not get you where you want to go. Holistic well-being is a group effort. A team sport, if you will.

At various points in writing this book, I have found myself stuck and unsure of what to do next. In one case, I was coming up empty on older Gardeners to interview and needed help drumming up interest. I put out a call to my Facebook community and within two days, I had forty Black elders from all over the country, ready and willing to sit down with me and talk. Another time, I had the worst case of writer's block. I let my community know and again, within days, I had two cowriting sessions scheduled, one voice note from a friend with a visualization exercise, and another friend who simply wanted to "lay eyes" on me and pray me into a more creative space.

That type of vulnerability ("I don't know how to move forward") is relatively new for me, but it has made the road ahead so much lighter and easier to navigate. I'm slowly but surely learning what it means to walk through life hand in hand with my community. When I walked through life holding people at arm's length, I felt safe but alone. I didn't trust people to catch me or hold space for me in my low moments, even when I would make it a point to be there in their low moments. I never gave people the opportunity to return the favor. I had to understand that love is a two-way street. You have to give *and* receive. Learning to stretch your hand out and hope that another person grasps it has been the biggest lesson of my life.

LET IT BE EASY

A FEW YEARS AGO, during one of our twice monthly therapy sessions, my therapist cleared her throat and laid a proposition in front of me.

"What if you leaned back a little bit?"

I didn't follow. "Lean back?"

"Yes."

We had spent the previous sessions talking about how tired I was. My loneliness was becoming more apparent, and I wasn't feeling sufficiently supported in many areas of my life.

I also shared how I tend to be proactive and engaged and considerate. I'm that friend who remembers the details. I check in if I notice you're quieter or more preoccupied than usual. I like to resolve conflict and am big on direct communication. If there's something I want, I'm speaking up about it. If I have a goal in mind, I am willing to work hard—to sacrifice!—to make it happen.

She asked me to consider what would happen if I just . . . didn't?

What would happen if I paused before immediately responding to emails?

What would happen if I didn't take the lead on repair conversations with my husband? If I waited for friends to invite *me* to brunch? If I stopped worrying about how everybody else was feeling and focused almost solely on how I was feeling?

I wish I could describe the frustration and resistance that built up inside me. I was furious. I *like* being the connector among my friends. I am *intentional* about my life. I am a *go-getter.*

Sit back? What is she even talking about?

But my promise to myself in therapy is that whatever my therapist suggests, I try it on first to see if it fits before discarding it completely. As I relaxed and let her words penetrate, I recognized the wisdom.

Sometimes I've been so busy playing gardener that if I paused for a minute, I might notice some of the gardens I'm tending are actually dead.

I can attribute my behaviors to any number of things: anxiety, my perfectionism, my eldest daughter upbringing, my all-girls Catholic high school conditioning that "women can do anything!," my ten plus years of entrepreneurship, my literal DNA from generations of women who knew shit had to get done so they rolled up their sleeves and did it themselves.

What she was suggesting: I can sit back and relax. Everything doesn't require me to be in charge. Allow others in my life to show up authentically, and either love them or leave them where they are. Where I recognize an area has fallen short of my needs, then I can do the work to fix it. I don't have to constantly be on guard. (There goes that anxiety again.)

I sat back. Here's what happened:

I held off on my "hey, just checking in" texts. My closest friends checked in to see how I was doing and within two weeks I got invites for coffee, breakfast, and a hike. I also took the time to recognize that a few relationships I had been holding dear were past their expiration date.

My husband took me on a date unexpectedly and later took over the travel arrangements for our upcoming trip, including making an honest-to-God agenda that he printed and gave me a copy of two days before we left.

I restarted my fitness journey. I spent thirty minutes a day, nearly every day, lifting weights and moving. It gave me such mental clarity and it felt like a little gift I gave myself every morning.

I stopped hovering over my inbox. I got an invite for a speaking engagement one week in. They paid the invoice three days later. Glory!

I'm still soaking in the lesson of letting good things come to me. Not feeling so anxious and panicky about what will happen but allowing the natural rhythms of life to unfold.

In a few short words she gave me permission to make my life about me again. *It's me season.* Worth every bit of that co-pay.

Do we always have to fight for the things we want? Is there any room for the journey to be, dare I say it . . . easy? We may be suspicious when things are "too easy" and instead of simply enjoying whatever has fallen into our lap, we're waiting for the other shoe to drop. If we have a lifetime of evidence that hustle and stress come before any good thing, then it makes sense that we feel we have to fight for our wins.

But what if good and easy and lovely could be our default? What would that feel like? Do you, anywhere in your mind, feel like it's possible? To me, ease feels like a hammock. Resting in the knowledge that you're supported. You don't have to hold yourself up alone. I encourage you to make friends with ease. (Or, in some cases, let ease make friends with you.)

SIMPLE SHIFTS

AUTHORS AND RESEARCHERS Emily and Amelia Nagoski suggest that 42 percent of your day be devoted to rest.[1] *Forty-two percent.* Science has shown that roughly ten hours a day devoted to the upkeep of self gives you the best chance at maintaining your well-being. Anything less than that for a significant amount of time and you're headed for trouble. As the authors warn, "If you don't find time for that 42 percent, that 42 percent will find you."

Forty-two percent is roughly ten hours each day. To hit the goal, start with hours of sleep (eight is perhaps ideal for you) and add in a couple more hours to get to your ten. These two hours will become the backbone of your consistent self-care practice.

So how should you structure your day so you can make sure you're always at the top of your list? It's the top question women ask me when joining our community and my answer is simple:

A.M. P.M.

In the morning, do something for yourself. In the evening, do something for yourself.

Easy. Done.

I've followed this system (can I even call it a system when it's so damn easy?) for close to ten years now.

It's the simplest thing I can think of to make sure I don't lose sight of who I am and what I need to thrive in a world that pulls on me damn near every waking moment.

Proving there is nothing new under the sun and the simplest solutions are best, a few Gardeners had implemented a form of the A.M./P.M. system to help structure their self-care practices.

Ifetayo White, 79, of South Carolina, shared that she started forty years ago when her daughters were 12 and 9. In 1982, White was a newly single mother, living in Washington, DC, when she confided to a friend that she couldn't get her mind to stop racing. That friend suggested she try meditation. Desperate for some kind of mental calm and clarity, she committed to twenty minutes in the morning and twenty minutes in the early evening. The morning effort, she realized, was the easy part. Finding twenty minutes during the after-school period was harder to implement.

"I knew inside of myself, I had to do something to shift myself from being a working woman out in the world to being a mom, to cook dinner, to have to listen to homework," White told me. "My children were of course very upset about that initially, knocking on the door. 'Cause I said, under no circumstances are you to interrupt me unless somebody is dying. They would be whispering under the door, knocking on the door, *Mommy, Mama, Mom*. But spirit was strong in me because I just kept saying, I have to do this for myself to be able to be gracious and not angry with my children for the rest of the day."

White found her way. Over the course of that year, it "changed my whole everything," she said. She became a believer in not only meditation but shifting the expectations placed on her and other Black women.

"It's an act of courage to say, I need ten minutes just to go in my room and close the door. You know what I'm saying? Because you have somebody waiting to eat or somebody needs you to drive them to the gym. But we have to start with one small step of courage for ourselves and realize that every time I take that step, I am shifting the generational lie that I'm on this earth to take care of everybody before myself, before my own needs."

White and I continued chatting for what felt like forever but really was just shy of an hour. But her "one small step of courage" comment immediately imprinted on me. That's what the A.M./P.M. routine is. It's a commitment to *you*, every day, every time.

What this routine does is twofold: It powers you up for whatever your day has in store for you. You get in some me-time before work, before traffic, before kids, before whatever stresses pop up in your day. Then, it releases whatever stress you may have accumulated during the day so you can rest and replenish yourself before bed.

As I've said before, there is no one on the planet tasked with ensuring you have a good day. That is why it is so crucial for you to be that person for yourself. For you to be the one who stops and asks, *What do I need? And how can I get it?*

First, there are three questions you have to ask yourself: *What's accessible (for me)? What's affordable (for me)? What's affirming (for me)?* I add that parenthetical because it's important to focus on what *you* like, and not what folks tell you should be a part of your self-care routine (not even me). It doesn't have to be social media worthy or even particularly beautiful.

ACCESSIBLE

Accessible simply means that it is not difficult for you to have access. It doesn't require a two-hour commute or any prohibitively expensive equipment. It's you and the things you have on hand or could reasonably have on hand at any given moment. What may be accessible is hot water and a tub. Or hot water and a tea bag. Or a good book.

AFFORDABLE

The cheapest forms of self-care fill me up most—a phone call with a friend, a walk in the sun, a forty-five-minute nap. I don't believe that you must spend money to take care of yourself. All those fancy room sprays and aromatherapy soaks have their place, but when it comes to self-care, I frequently think in terms of $20 or less. Or better yet, free.

AFFIRMING

What's affirming to me are things that appeal to my senses. I love things that make me feel good in my own skin, give me a sense of calm and ground me when I'm feeling off-balance. For that reason, I love a few good playlists for my different moods, I love smell goods, and I love a good meal. You know that mix of joy and anticipation you get when you see the waiter bringing your food? That's the feeling you're aiming for.

LOOKING AT THESE three considerations, build your morning routine. In between the time you wake up and noon (or whatever your "morning" is, for second and third shift folks), add one thing that will set the tone for the day ahead.

Your morning routine could look like this:

6:00 a.m. Wake up + turn on your "Good Morning" playlist
6:15 a.m. Get some tea and sit in silence for a minute, mentally clearing out space for the day to come. (Or do some yoga stretches or dance to your favorite song or . . .)

7:00 a.m. Shower, get dressed, prep for the day ahead

7:30 a.m. Leave the house

It's not about creating elaborate routines that you have to do in the same exact order every single morning. It's about clearing out space to add an affirming, affordable, accessible activity to your day.

In the evening, consider it in the reverse. What do you need in those quiet moments before bed to get the day's stress off you? I hardly ever go to bed without some type of aromatherapy. I rotate between body butters and oils from Black-owned businesses and give myself a mini massage every night. It's my way of saying thank you to my body for getting me through another day.

Now, what might the A.M./P.M. system look like in practice for you?

A.M.	P.M.
Yoga/simple stretches Morning tea/coffee Journaling Mirror affirmations Prayer Music Silence (Underrated!!) Warm shower A delicious breakfast	Warm bath Self-massage with warm massage oil Reading Journaling Meditation Prayer Aromatherapy Calling/chatting with a friend

And really, this is just what *my* list looks like. These are activities I can turn to again and again to set the mood I desire.

Now, it's important for you to note that this is not the total of my self-care practice. This is the baseline. These are the activities I include in my day that are just as common and routine as brushing my teeth or washing my face.

Take a few minutes now to consider:

What can I add to my morning routine that fills me up? Am I a downward dog person or a long bath person? How much time can I devote to myself each morning? What can I add to my evening routine that soothes me? What time do I need to start winding down each evening to ensure I get adequate rest?

No matter what you select, if it's grounded in what's affirming, affordable, and accessible to you, you can't lose.

CREATE A CARE GUIDE

ANYTIME YOU GET a new plant, you spend time learning its care needs. If you buy from a reputable garden center or plant store, they'll have instructions tucked into the plant to make it easy for you. You don't have to guess how much light it needs or how often to water. They spell it out for you. Where that instruction is missing, you then have to Google or ask a more knowledgeable plant parent what to do and when to do it.

When it comes to you, dear reader, I want that knowledge of how to care for you to be just that simple.

I'm challenging you to write a care guide for yourself, so that anyone who wishes to know how to care for you best can know exactly how much light and how much water you need. The best way forward is to understand who you are, what you need, and where those needs will be met. That's it. It's a fairly simple process but due to life's ever-increasing complexity, we make it seem harder than it truly is.

During a particularly challenging time of my life, where I had more needs than supportive ways to meet them, I wrote this care guide to help those who loved me understand the best way to show up. Just the act of writing soothed me greatly. Use mine as a template to craft your own.

TPJ CARE GUIDE

This is a living, breathing document that captures what I know about myself, at 37 years old. All those who care for me and want me to be the best version of myself should know these things. Some items may appear contradictory or perhaps illogical. But I accept that and note it anyway.

When I'm sad

Find me a quiet place to be. Let me put my head in your lap and stroke my hair. Rub your hands firmly up and down my spine. Hug me. Hold me. Check to see if I have eaten. If I have not eaten, feed me. If I tell you I don't have an appetite, get me a bowl of rice with butter and salt. I will always eat a bowl of rice with butter and salt. Give me at least thirty minutes of your time. An hour would be more ideal.

When I'm overwhelmed

Please affirm the overwhelm. Take important stock of the areas of my life that are heavy. I need to put them down. Step in where you can. If you don't know how to step in, just watch what I do and then step in. Place a magazine on my lap and a glass of ice water on the side table.

When I'm struggling to be vulnerable

Show me the way. Be patient with me. Vulnerability is not the easiest area for me to access. I have years of practice keeping things close to my chest, solving most of my problems internally. Please allow me to practice being soft and open with you.

When my anxiety flares

Remind me that I am loved. Remind me that my brain does not get to decide how things end up. Remind me to move, to shake, to twirl, to spin. Remind me to release what's not mine to carry.

When I don't feel loved

Tell me you love me. Add in the "why" for a little razzle-dazzle.

When I am tired

Allow me to rest without wondering how long I will rest. Allow me to be still. Wrap your arms around me and squeeze gently.

When I'm having a great day

Join in my joy with me. Ask questions. Ask a follow-up question. Allow me to gush and be thrilled. Remind me that this joy is hard-earned and I deserve it.

When I'm unusually quiet

Sometimes there's no reason for it but sometimes there is. I promise to try my best to be open about it but if you can, please ask, "Is there anything you want to talk about?"

When I'm struggling to make a decision

Remind me of my wisdom. Let me figure out the best path forward and tell me you'll be there to support me either way.

IF YOU ARE unsure about where to start with your care guide, picture this: You have your best friend in the world with you, whether that's a platonic love or a romantic one. You are 100 percent sure about their desire and capacity to help you. There is nothing they won't do for you. You lack any hesitation or insecurities. You know you deserve the level of care they want to give you. They are asking you, "What will help at this moment?"

This care guide is your best answer.

Sometimes *you* will be the person responding to your needs and giving yourself care. And how lovely will it feel when you are able to show up for yourself exactly how you need it.

We all get sad. We all get overwhelmed. We all get tired. What should happen when those things occur? Much of our stress and unhappiness comes not because of the misalignments in life, but because we don't know what to do when they come.

In writing what you need, you give yourself permission to receive it. That may be foreign to you, after a lifetime of shrinking from your needs. But being needy is part of the human condition. Your needs exist and should be met.

STAND IN THE SUN

AS I TYPE THIS, my daughter is roughly one month from stepping foot on her first-choice college campus, a bright-eyed aspiring screenwriter. (Full transparency: I typed most of this book through tears as I thought about my eldest leaving the nest.)

It is not lost on me as I write this book about Black women and lessons on wellness they've learned from their mothers, that I am praying my lessons have landed in her heart as I intended. I'm launching my daughter, my oldest baby, into a world that frightens me, but these feelings are no different from the feelings my mother faced, or her mother, or her mother. All we can do is reaffirm our commitment to loving our children, wherever they reside, being the sun and water to their seeds.

After talking to one hundred women, including my mother and grandmother, there was only one more I needed to talk to: my daughter. This letter is the result of everything I know and hold dear.

Dear Daughter,

I hope you know that I love you tremendously. I hope there is not a doubt in your mind that I have tried to surround you and your brother with as much love as you can stand.

I hope I've told you that you deserve the world. That you deserve to take up space, to be bold, to use your voice, to chase whatever dream you desire. I hope you understand that you have been blessed with many gifts and however you decide to express yourself creatively, it will fuel you.

I hope you've learned from me how to prioritize your mental and emotional health so you can be the woman you want to grow into. Stay in places that feel warm and good to your soul.

I hope I have given you a solid spiritual foundation that

you can take and shape as your own. I hope you know your place in this world is divinely ordained.

I hope you enter adulthood with a good understanding of how to take care of your body, the vessel that allows everything to happen. Listen intently to any signals your body is giving you, including the soft hum in your gut that something isn't right.

I hope I've given you good, solid examples of female friendship so you know what good platonic love looks like when you see it. I hope that your father and I have shown you how to navigate healthy long-term partnership, and you understand how to voice your needs.

I hope I've taught you how to pursue professional spaces where you don't have to shout or cry to be heard. I hope I have given you an example of what it means to tend to yourself in every season.

I hope I taught you that your worth isn't found in your exhaustion. I hope I reminded you how to wield your strength in a way that helps, not harms, you.

I haven't always gotten it right (there are definitely some weeds in your garden I allowed in) but know that I tried my absolute best to make the main things the main things. As you emerge in adulthood, I hope you are surrounded by people who love you and inspire you to love yourself harder.

I hope I taught you that you deserve to stand in the sun.

Here (always) to see you bloom,
Mummy

ACKNOWLEDGMENTS

I WANT TO thank 17-year-old me. This entire book is for you.

I want to thank God for placing me in the right place at the right time with the right people so this book could exist. To my editors Makayla Tabron and Abby West: Thank you for your endless encouragement and sharp editing to make this book sing. To Kristina Sutton Lennon, the best literary agent I could have asked for. You believed in this project so fully from day one and helped me land at a dream of a publishing house. Thank you, thank you. To all my writer friends, thank you for showing me how it's done, especially L'Oreal for holding my hand during the pitching process and reminding me that I didn't need to complete a perfect first draft. To Amber for just being the best friend to me over the last decade. To Da'Shika for our walks to clear our mind and find our footing. I have too many friends and supporters to name individually but know that you were instrumental in keeping my mind sharp and my thoughts cohesive.

To my family, especially my sisters, thank you for always believing that my writing was something worth reading. To my parents, I appreciate every drop you've poured into me. I can't thank you enough. To my kids, I am so thankful to be your mother. Writing this book while preparing to launch you into adulthood was such a delicate balance but I pray I did it well. If anyone asks what's the greatest part of my life, it's you. To my husband, you've always been my biggest cheerleader. Thank you for getting me to the finish line.

Finally, I need to acknowledge the Gardeners, the women who gave me time and insight into their lives. Thank you for sharing this process with me and allowing us to learn from you. May you continue to bloom in delightful and unexpected ways.

a'driane nieves
Akirah Wyatt
Alecia Velma Jackson
Alisha Robertson
Andrea Ranae Johnson
Andree Miller
Aneesha McGregor
Angela Holliday-Bell
Angelique Dyer
Ashantis Jones
Ashleigh Vaughn
Assia Lauren
Barbara Earle
Barbara Johnson
Bertha H. Brown
Brandi Denise Boyd
Britney Minor
Bronlynn Thurman
Carlise Cartwright
Chakayla Taylor
Chana Timms
Charlotte Edwards
Christyna Johnson
Claire Dorsey
Colette Hill
Courtney Clayton Jenkins
Cynthia Moore
Da'Shika Street
Danielle Finney
Danyelle Thomas
Dawn M. Rivers
Denise Brown
Deveter Brown
Dionne Stalling
Eryka Parker
Essie Gilchrist
Esther Boykin
Felicia Hopkins
Frechic Burton
Gloria Clifton
Habeebah Grimes
Halleemah Nash
Ifetayo White
India Pierce
Janay Jefferson
Jeryl Legions
Jessica Travis
Kara Stevens
Karla Simpson
Kat Vellos

Kimberly Young
Kristen Jeffers
Krystal Pollard-Reddick
L'Oreal Thompson Payton
Lakeshia Poole
Latorsha Peake
Laura Farris-Daughtery
Lauren Henderson
Lauren Wilson
Liz King
Lois McClendon
Lorrie Gates
Louise Moody
Lyvonne Briggs
Marcie Thomas
Marilyn Williams Pringle
Maudie M. Murray
Melissa Kimble
Michelle Smith
Michelle Starling
Nadirah Habeebullah
Nailah Blades
Naj Austin
Natalyn Bradshaw
Natasha Nicholes
Necole Gibson
Nike Olabisi-Green
Nikki Carpenter
Nikki Porcher
Olivia Lauer
Pamela Combs
Pamela Davis
Reesheeda Graham Washington
Rogena Burrus
Saisha Baskerville
Samantha Saunders
Shamell Roberts
Stacey Jeffries
Stephanie Armstrong
Stephanie Ghoston Paul
Stephanie Perry
Sylvia Johnson
Talise Campbell
Taya Dunn Johnson
Teka Johnson
Ursula Foster
Valencia Joy
Vanessa Goodar
Vickie Nichols
Vicky Butler
Yetti Ojayi-Obe
Zinga Hart

Notes

1 Black Wellness Matters

1. CDC, National Vital Statistics Report, Vol. 69, No. 13, Table 10, www.cdc.gov/nchs/data/nvsr/nvsr69/nvsr69-13-508.pdf.

2. *The Atlantic*, "The Racial Inequality of Sleep," www.theatlantic.com/health/archive/2015/10/the-sleep-gap-and-racial-inequality/412405/.

3. "Black/African American," NAMI, October 15, 2024, www.nami.org/your-journey/identity-and-cultural-dimensions/black-african-american/.

4. *Human Nature*, March 2010, www.ncbi.nlm.nih.gov/pmc/articles/PMC2861506/.

5. Heather Dockray, "Self-Care Isn't Enough: We Need Community Care to Thrive," Mashable, May 24, 2019, mashable.com/article/community-care-versus-self-care.

6. AFROPUNKTV, "Radical Self Care: Angela Davis," YouTube, December 17, 2018, www.youtube.com/watch?v=Q1cHoL4vaBs.

7. Emily Nagoski and Amelia Nagoski, *Burnout: The Secret to Unlocking the Stress Cycle*, paperback ed. (Ballantine Books, 2020), 27.

2 Coming Home to Our Bodies: Physical Wellness

1. "#KeepItDown Confederate Flag Takedown," YouTube, The Tribe CLT, June 27, 2015, www.youtube.com/watch?v=gr-mt1P94cQ.

2. #teamEBONY, "[In My Lifetime] Bree Newsome on Removing the Confederate Battle Flag," *Ebony*, February 5, 2016, www.ebony.com/bree-newsome-confederate-flag-ebonybhm/.

3. Emily Nagoski and Amelia Nagoski, *Burnout: The Secret to Unlocking the Stress Cycle*, 1st ed. (Ballantine Books, 2019).

4. Jessamyn Stanley, *Yoke: My Yoga of Self-Acceptance*. (Workman, 2021).

5. Cody Short, "New Groups Are Changing the Narrative about Black Women and the Outdoors," NPR, February 7, 2023, www.npr.org/2023/02/07/1155186965/new-groups-are-changing-the-narrative-about-black-women-and-the-outdoors.

6. Matthew P. Walker, *Why We Sleep: Unlocking the Power of Sleep and Dreams* (Scribner, an Imprint of Simon & Schuster, 2018).

7. Benjamin Reiss, "Op-Ed: African Americans Don't Sleep as Well as Whites, an

Inequality Stretching Back to Slavery," *Los Angeles Times*, April 23, 2017, www.latimes.com/opinion/op-ed/la-oe-reiss-race-sleep-gap-20170423-story.html.

8. A. M. Williamson and A. M. Feyer, "Moderate Sleep Deprivation Produces Impairments in Cognitive and Motor Performance Equivalent to Legally Prescribed Levels of Alcohol Intoxication," *Occupational and Environmental Medicine* 57, no. 10 (October 2000): 649–55. doi: 10.1136/oem.57.10.649; PMID: 10984335; PMCID: PMC1739867.

9. Light Watkins, *Bliss More: How to Succeed in Meditation without Really Trying* (Ballantine Books, 2018).

10. Ev'Yan Whitney, *Sensual Self: Prompts and Practices for Getting in Touch with Your Body* (Clarkson Potter, 2021).

11. Amy Wallace, "Viola Davis as You've Never Seen Her Before: Leading Lady!" *New York Times*, September 12, 2014, www.nytimes.com/2014/09/14/magazine/viola-davis.html.

12. Jennifer Wright Knust, *Unprotected Texts: The Bible's Surprising Contradictions about Sex and Desire* (HarperCollins, 2011).

13. Ashley Townes et al., "Partnered Sexual Behaviors, Pleasure, and Orgasms at Last Sexual Encounter: Findings from a U.S. Probability Sample of Black Women Ages 18 to 92 Years," *Journal of Sex & Marital Therapy* 47, no. 4 (2021): 353–67. doi:10.1080/0092623X.2021.1878315.

3 Our Friends, Ourselves: Social Wellness

1. "Oprah Winfrey & Gayle King on 46 Years of Friendship: 'No Matter What, I'm Here for You,'" YouTube, *People* magazine, April 26, 2022, www.youtube.com/watch?v=GHgL6yvR0to.

2. "Live from the NYPL: Toni Morrison and Junot Diaz," New York Public Library, December 13, 2013, www.nypl.org/audiovideo/toni-morrison-junot-d%C3%ADaz.

3. Pyar Seth, "Nikki Giovanni on Rest, Love, and Care," Public Books, October 12, 2021, www.publicbooks.org/nikki-giovanni-on-rest-love-and-care/.

4. "Loneliness and Its Impact on the American Workplace—Cigna Healthcare," accessed May 24, 2023. www.cigna.com/static/www-cigna-com/docs/about-us/newsroom/studies-and-reports/combatting-loneliness/loneliness-and-its-impact-on-the-american-workplace.pdf.

5. "The Loneliness Epidemic Persists: A Post-Pandemic Look at the State of Loneliness among U.S. Adults," The Cigna Group Newsroom, 2022, https://newsroom.thecignagroup.com/loneliness-epidemic-persists-post-pandemic-look.

6. "Social Connection—Current Priorities of the U.S. Surgeon General," n.d., www.hhs.gov/surgeongeneral/priorities/connection/index.html.

7. E. C. Bronder, S. L. Speight, K. M. Witherspoon, and A. J. Thomas, "John Henryism, Depression, and Perceived Social Support in Black Women," *Journal of Black Psychology* 40 (2013): 115–37. doi:10.1177/0095798412474466.

8. Jasmine A. Abrams, Morgan Maxwell, Michell Pope, and Faye Z. Belgrave, "Carrying the World with the Grace of a Lady and the Grit of a Warrior," *Psychology of Women Quarterly* 38, no. 4 (2014): 503–18. https://doi.org/10.1177/0361684314541418.

9. Chanequa Walker-Barnes, "When the Bough Breaks: The StrongBlackWoman and the Embodiment of Stress," in *Black Women's Mental Health: Balancing Strength and Vulnerability*, ed. Stephanie Y. Evans, Kanika Bell, and Nsenga K. Burton (State University of New York Press, 2018).

10. Natalie N. Watson-Singleton, "Strong Black Woman Schema and Psychological Distress: The Mediating Role of Perceived Emotional Support," *Journal of Black Psychology* 43, no. 8 (2017): 778–88. https://doi.org/10.1177/0095798417732414.

11. C. L. Woods-Giscombé, "Superwoman Schema: African American Women's Views on Stress, Strength, and Health," *Qualitative Health Research* 20 (2010): 668–83.

12. J. Holt-Lunstad, "Why Social Relationships Are Important for Physical Health: A Systems Approach to Understanding and Modifying Risk and Protection," *Annual Review of Psychology* 69 (2018): 437–58.

13. Joshua Moreton, Caitlin S. Kelly, and Gillian M. Sandstrom, "Social Support from Weak Ties: Insight from the Literature on Minimal Social Interactions," *Social and Personality Psychology Compass* (January 2023), doi:10.1111/spc3.12729.

14. Brene Brown, *Daring Greatly: How the Courage to Be Vulnerable Transforms the Way We Live, Love, Parent* (Garamond Press, 2012).

15. K. Vellos, "The Hidden Barrier to Finding Your Third Place and How to Overcome It," We Should Get Together, March 1, 2024, https://weshouldgettogether.com/blog/hidden-barrier-to-third-place-and-how-to-overcome-it.

16. L. Kroencke, G. M. Harari, M. D. Back, and J. Wagner, "Well-Being in Social Interactions: Examining Personality-Situation Dynamics in Face-to-Face and Computer-Mediated Communication," *Journal of Personality and Social Psychology* 124, no. 2 (2023):437–60.

4 Carving Our Own Lanes: Professional Wellness

1. "Negro Women to Be Put to Work," *Newspapers.com*, October 2, 1918, www.newspapers.com/article/the-greenville-news-negro-women-to-be-pu/38314573/?locale=en-US.

2. Cindy Hahamovitch, *The Fruits of Their Labor: Atlantic Coast Farmworkers and*

the Making of Migrant Poverty, 1870–1945 (University of North Carolina Press, 1997).

3. "Records of Rights," NAACP Telegram Regarding Forced Labor of Women, 1918, recordsofrights.org/records/280/naacp-telegram-regarding-forced-labor-of-women, accessed January 25, 2024.

4. Katherine R. Allen and Victoria Chin-Sang, "A Lifetime of Work: The Context and Meanings of Leisure for Aging Black Women," *The Gerontologist* 30, no. 6 (December 1990): 734–40, https://doi.org/10.1093/geront/30.6.734.

5. Madeline Garfinkle, "Want a Higher Salary? Job Hopping Boosts Pay, per New Report," *Entrepreneur,* September 6, 2024, https://entm.ag/C41kXu.

6. Pauline Rose Clance and Suzanne Ament Imes, "The Imposter Phenomenon in High Achieving Women: Dynamics and Therapeutic Intervention," *Psychotherapy: Theory, Research & Practice* 15, no. 3 (1978): 241.

7. Pearl Cleage, *Things I Should Have Told My Daughter: Lies, Lessons, and Love Affairs* (Atria Books, 2014).

8. "Twice as Hard: Overqualified Black Women Need to Protect Themselves at Work," YouTube, All Things Equitable, February 22, 2022, youtu.be/9hz3td0_ozA?si=5E1i2LLTowFhfkCi.

9. "So Be It, See to It: From the Archives of Octavia Butler," *Paris Review,* March 23, 2018, www.theparisreview.org/blog/2018/03/23/so-be-it-see-to-it-from-the-archives-of-octavia-butler/.

10. Elena Dure, "Black Women Are the Fastest Growing Group of Entrepreneurs, But the Job Isn't Easy," J. P. Morgan, October 21, 2021, www.jpmorgan.com/insights/business/business-planning/black-women-are-the-fastest-growing-group-of-entrepreneurs-but-the-job-isnt-easy.

11. Dure, "Black Women Are the Fastest Growing Group of Entrepreneurs."

12. Dure, "Black Women Are the Fastest Growing Group of Entrepreneurs."

13. Dure, "Black Women Are the Fastest Growing Group of Entrepreneurs."

14. Arlan Hamilton, "Why Are Underrepresented Founders Still Not Getting Venture Capital Funding?" Mashable, February 27, 2023, mashable.com/article/arlan-hamilton-black-founders-vc-backstage-capital.

15. Brian Wong, "This Actress and Writer Just Offered 1 Piece of Simple but Powerful Networking Advice," Inc, October 20, 2017, www.inc.com/brian-wong/this-actress-writer-just-offered-1-piece-of-simple-but-powerful-networking-advice.html.

5 Fill Me Up: Spiritual Wellness

1. "Religious Beliefs Among Black Americans," Pew Research Center's Religion and Public Life Project, Pew Research Center, February 16, 2021, www.pewresearch.org/religion/2021/02/16/religious-beliefs-among-black-americans/.

2. "In U.S., Decline of Christianity Continues at Rapid Pace," Pew Research Center's Religion and Public Life Project, Pew Research Center, October 17, 2019, www.pewresearch.org/religion/2019/10/17/in-u-s-decline-of-christianity-continues-at-rapid-pace/.

3. C. Y. Wiley, "The Intersection of Religion and Mental Well-Being amongst African-American Women," *Journal of Religion and Spirituality in Social Work: Social Thought* 39, no. 3 (2020): 225–247. https://doi.org/10.1080/15426432.2020.1784070.

4. Alice Walker, *In Search of Our Mothers' Gardens: Womanist Prose* (Harcourt Brace Jovanovich, 1983).

5. "Your Grandmother's Theology," *U.S. Catholic*, May 2023, 20–24.

6. Eileen Campbell-Reed, "State of Clergywomen in the United States: A Statistical Update," https://eileencampbellreed.org/state-of-clergy/.

7. Zora Neale Hurston, *Their Eyes Were Watching God* (Perennial Classics, 1937).

8. Kristin Neff, *Self-Compassion: The Proven Power of Being Kind to Yourself* (Hodder & Stoughton, 2013).

9. Tiya Miles, "When Everyone around You Is Talking about the End, Talk about Black History," *New York Times*, February 13, 2022, www.nytimes.com/2022/02/13/opinion/apocalyptic-thinking-black-history.html.

10. John Mark Comer and John Ortberg, *The Ruthless Elimination of Hurry: Staying Emotionally Healthy and Spiritually Alive in Our Current Chaos* (WaterBrook, 2019).

11. D. Danyelle Thomas, "Dear Church Folk: I Wish Y'all Would Stfu about Ancestor Veneration," *Unfit Christian*, August 21, 2020, www.unfitchristian.com/ancestor-veneration/.

12. Camille T. Dungy, *Soil: The Story of a Black Mother's Garden* (Simon & Schuster, 2023).

6 Settling Our Nerves: Mental and Emotional Wellness

1. Susan L. Taylor, *All About Love: Favorite Selections from in the Spirit; On Living Fearlessly* (Urban Books, 2008).

2. "Depression May Look Different in Black Women," NYU, December 13, 2022, www.nyu.edu/about/news-publications/news/2022/december/depression-Black-women.html.

3. American Psychological Association, 2022, Demographics of U.S. Psychology Workforce [Interactive data tool], www.apa.org/workforce/data-tools/demographics.

4. "Equity, Diversity and Inclusion," American Psychological Association, www.apa.org/about/apa/equity-diversity-inclusion, accessed April 10, 2024.

5. Nancy Gillen, "Reese Witherspoon Tells Tracee Ellis Ross How She Conquered Hollywood," *Interview Magazine*, June 15, 2021, www.interviewmagazine.com/film/reese-witherspoon-tells-tracee-ellis-ross-how-she-conquered-hollywood.

6. "Anger: The Black Woman's 'Superpower,'" NPR, May 15, 2019, www.npr.org/transcripts/723322372.

7. Inger Burnett-Zeigler, *Nobody Knows the Trouble I've Seen: The Emotional Lives of Black Women* (Amistad, 2022).

8. bell hooks, *All About Love: New Visions* (William Morrow, an Imprint of HarperCollins Publishers, 2022).

7 Honoring Our Creativity: Creative Wellness

1. Melissa Kimble, "The Story behind the Billboard X 'Higher,'" Songs in the Key of Community by Melissa Kimble, November 10, 2023, melissakimble.sustack.com/p/the-story-behind-the-billboard-x?utm_source=profile&utm_medum=reader.

2. Nikki Giovanni, *The Prosaic Soul of Nikki Giovanni* (HarperCollins e-Books, 2014).

3. Kimber Thomas, "Makeshifting: Black Women and Resilient Creativity in the Rural South," *Southern Cultures* 26 no. 1 (2020): 120–37. Project MUSE, https://dx.doi.org/10.1353/scu.2020.000.

4. "Lucille Clifton: Interview," *Mosaic Literary Magazine*, April 6, 2023, mosaimagazine.org/lucille-clifton-interview.

5. Alice Walker, *In Search of Our Mothers' Gardens: Womanist Prose* (Mariner Books, 2003).

6. Kate Rix, "How Much Recess Should Kids Get?," *U.S. News and World Report*, October 2022, www.usnews.com/education/k12/articles/how-much-recess-should-kids-get.

7. The Galavanting Bae, Nicole Goss, www.instagram.com/theegalavantingbae/.

8. Patia Braithwaite, "In Praise of Black People Laughing," *SELF*, June 23, 2020, www.self.com/story/black-people-laughing.

9. "Nina Simone: To Be Free," YouTube, February 2013, www.youtube.com/watch?v=Si5uW6cnyG4.

10. Ruha Benjamin, *Imagination: A Manifesto* (W. W. Norton, 2024).

11. a'driane nieves, https://www.instagram.com/p/COVHx8bl8Ne/, accessed August 15, 2025.

8 In Full Bloom

1. Nagoski and Nagoski, *Burnout*.

ABOUT THE AUTHOR

TARA PRINGLE JEFFERSON is the founder of The Self Care Suite, a digital wellness community for Black women. Over the last decade, Jefferson has brought her wellness expertise to corporate audiences including WW, SiriusXM, Wayfair, and Priceline. Her voice has been featured on *New York* magazine's *The Cut*, *Black Enterprise*, and *Essence*. When she's not writing, she finds peace among her houseplants and flowers (even when they don't bloom). A Cleveland native, she lives in northeast Ohio with her husband and two children.